THE CORNEA

Publisher: Caroline Makepeace
Development editor: Myriam Brearley
Production Controller: Chris Jarvis
Desk editor: Claire Hutchins
Cover designer: Fred Rose

THE CORNEA:
its examination in contact lens practice

Edited by:

Nathan Efron
BScOptom PhD(Melbourne) DSc(UMIST) MCOptom FAAO(Dip CL)
FIACLE FCLSA FVCO MILT

Professor of Clinical Optometry
Director, European Centre for Contact Lens Research, Department of
Optometry and Neuroscience, University of Manchester Institute of Science
and Technology, Manchester, UK

Honorary Professor, Department of Ophthalmology, The University of
Manchester, Manchester, UK

Adjunct Professor, School of Optometry, Faculty of Health, Queensland
University of Technology, Brisbane, Australia

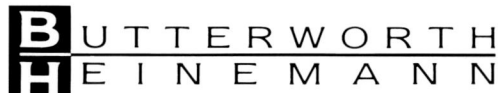

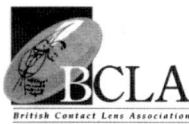

OXFORD   AUCKLAND   BOSTON   JOHANNESBURG   MELBOURNE   NEW DELHI

Butterworth-Heinemann
Linacre House, Jordan Hill, Oxford OX2 8DP
225 Wildwood Avenue, Woburn, MA 01801-2041
A division of Reed Educational and Professional Publishing Ltd

ℛ A member of the Reed Elsevier plc group

First published 2001

British Library Cataloguing in Publication Data
The cornea: its examination in contact lens practice
 1. Cornea – Examination 2. Contact lenses
 I. Efron, Nathan
 617.7'19

Library of Congress Cataloguing in Publication Data
A catalogue record for this book is available from the Library of Congress

ISBN 0 7506 4798 1

Composition by Genesis Typesetting, Laser Quay, Rochester, Kent
Printed and bound in Spain

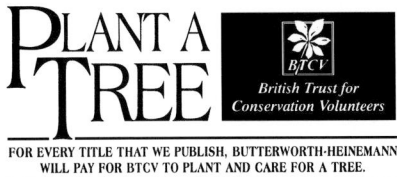

Contents List

Preface

In recent years, the British Contact Lens Association (BCLA) has been embarking upon an ambitious programme of hosting 'theme days' as part of its Annual Clinical Conference and Exhibition. The topic of the theme day held on Thursday 25 May 2000 in Birmingham, UK, was 'The Cornea: its Examination in Contact Lens Practice' – which of course is the title of this book. In essence, therefore, this book constitutes an expanded version of the transactions of that day.

I was delighted and honoured when the Conference Scientific Programme Officer of the BCLA – Jonathan Walker – invited me to act as moderator for the theme day. Our joint task was to help assemble an international team of eminent clinical scientists who were actively involved in research relating to examination of the structure of the cornea. Of course, there are many other aspects of the cornea that could have been considered – such as corneal physiology, pathology, immunology, molecular biology, refractive techniques, temperature, etc. – and there are various other ocular tissues that are affected by lens wear, such as the conjunctiva and eyelids. Perhaps various combinations of these topics will form the basis of future BCLA theme days (and long may they continue!). But our theme day was to be confined to the *examination* of the cornea in contact lens practice. Jonathan and I were delighted that all of the experts we 'targeted' for participation in the programme accepted our invitation and attended the conference. A photograph of the assembled speakers – taken during the lunchtime break on the day of the meeting – is featured at the end of this Preface. We are pictured standing in the same order (from left to right) as our respective chapters appear in this book.

At first glance, the restriction of the theme to the topic of corneal examination in contact lens practice may be considered by some to represent a 'back to basics' approach. After all, what could be more basic than examining the cornea of a contact lens wearer – a procedure that is the fundamental cornerstone of contact lens practice? In truth, of course, this topic is at the cutting edge of clinical technology. Advances in optical design, computer systems, video and digital image capture techniques, and image analysis software, have heralded the introduction of clinical instruments that can quickly and accurately facilitate tasks that we could only dream about a decade or so ago.

This book has been structured to progressively take the reader from the familiar clinical technique of slit lamp biomicroscopy – which can be used to obtain a general appraisal of the integrity of the cornea at relatively low magnification – through to increasingly sophisticated technologies of corneal examination. The topic of slit lamp biomicroscopy is so vast and of such immediate clinical relevance that the subject matter has been essentially divided into two parts. In Chapter 1, Lyndon Jones has drawn upon his unique blend of experience as both an award-winning clinician and active researcher, to produce an informative and authoritative overview of the techniques of using the slit lamp biomicroscope. This is a technique that we sometimes take for granted, but with our increasing knowledge of cornea–lens interactions, it is timely to review this topic so that we can exploit the slit lamp to its maximum potential. This chapter, which is co-authored by Deborah Jones – an accomplished clinical educator and practitioner – also covers the topic of the application of the slit lamp to examine non-sight-threatening complications of contact lens wear.

In Chapter 2, Barry Weissman and Bartly Mondino consider the slit lamp examination of the sight-threatening condition of microbial keratitis, and other related issues. Professor Weissman, a PhD-qualified optometrist, enjoys the privilege of holding a Chair in Ophthalmology in the prestigious Jules Stein Eye Institute at UCLA, and as such has had unrivalled access over many years to a vast cohort of patients suffering from contact lens-related infectious keratitis. Professors Weissman and Mondino have researched, published and lectured extensively on this topic, and all this experience is brought to bear in their thorough review of the presentation, risk factors, diagnosis and management of microbial keratitis as it relates to contact lens wear.

In 1997, my laboratory (Eurolens Research) was fortunate to acquire – through generous sponsorship from Bausch & Lomb – a Tomey P4 ConfoScan Slit Scanning Confocal Microscope, which was one of only about 25 such instruments deployed around the world at the time. A young and enthusiastic team of researchers (who we call the 'Confocal Team') came together to investigate the potential of this technique for understanding the response of the cornea to contact lens wear. Prior to the development of the clinical confocal microscope, the living cornea had never before been observed at a cellular level. It quickly became clear to us that entirely new paradigms for defining the normal and altered cornea needed to be developed, and that a long and fascinating research journey was lying in wait. But the time is now, and I am proud to be able to present in Chapter 3, together with my colleagues who constitute the Confocal Team, an account of our findings and thinking to date on this exciting topic.

Professor Jan Bergmanson has devoted the majority of his academic life to studies of the ultrastructure of the cornea in response to contact lens wear. He has approached this topic systematically, concentrating, at various stages of his career, on specific layers of the cornea. His writings constitute the standard references in the field. At this juncture in his career, Jan is perfectly placed to put together the various pieces of the 'corneal jigsaw'. Although the cornea is yet to be solved completely, Jan's succinct overview in Chapter 4 provides tremendous insights into the ultrastructure of normal cornea, and the way in which it responds and structurally adapts to the stress of contact lens wear.

Chapter 5 addresses the important question of corneal topography. This chapter is written by Professor Stephen Klyce, who is widely acknowledged as being the pioneer of modern corneal topographic analysis techniques. Although such instruments first became available over a decade ago, since then there have been tremendous advances that have vastly expanded the versatility and enhanced the utility of this methodology. Stephen Klyce has remained at the cutting edge of these advances, and his chapter will bring clinicians right up to date with respect to the latest developments in corneal topographic analysis, and the application of this technology to contact lens practice and refractive surgery.

It would be remiss of me not to acknowledge the existence of other technologies that can be used to image the cornea, but are not considered in this book. The logistical constraint of confining the themed event to a single day meant that there was no time to consider alternative and equally fascinating techniques such as optical coherence tomography, nuclear magnetic resonance imaging, and B-scan ultrasonography. The decision not to cover the above techniques in detail relates in part to the fact that very little research has been reported to date investigating the utility of these methodologies for examining the cornea in relation to contact lens wear. Nevertheless, it is important to recognize that alternative instruments are being developed and to appreciate that still better techniques may well emerge in the future for corneal examination.

I hope readers will enjoy this contemporary account of corneal examination during contact lens wear as much as I have enjoyed my task of editing this book.

Nathan Efron

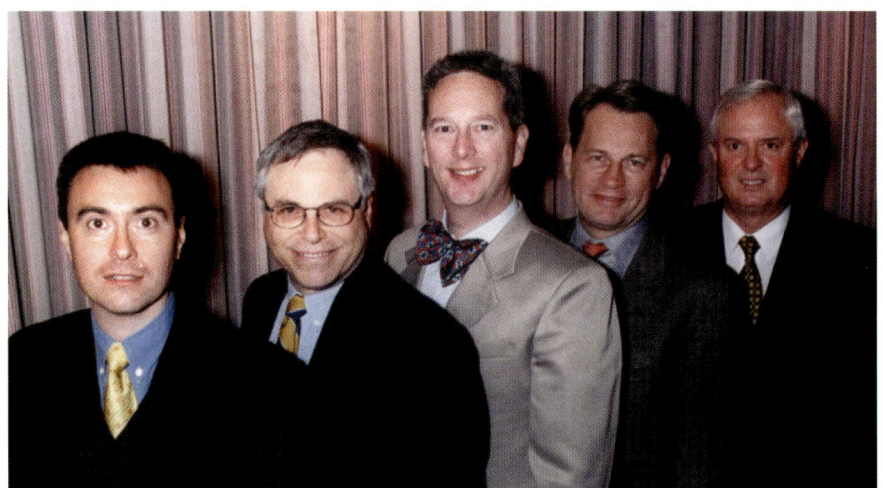

Presenters at the Cornea 'theme day', standing in the order that their chapters appear in this book (left to right): Lyndon Jones, Barry Weissman, Nathan Efron, Jan Bergmanson and Stephen Klyce.

Details of the Main Contributors

Chapter 1: Slit lamp biomicroscopy

Lyndon Jones is currently an Associate Professor at the University of Waterloo, Ontario, Canada. He graduated in Optometry from the University of Wales, Cardiff, in 1985 and worked as Research Optometrist at the Institute of Optometry in London up to 1992. Dr Jones then entered private practice, completing a part-time PhD at Aston University in 1998. He holds three of the higher awards granted by the British College of Optometrists, is a Fellow of the American Academy of Optometry, in which he is a Diplomate in Cornea and Contact Lenses, and is also a Fellow of the International Association of Contact Lens Educators. He is a former partner in a three times award-winning private practice in London and has been the recipient of a number of awards, including the *Optician* magazine's 'Contribution to Optics' Award (1996), the Peter Abel Award of the German Contact Lens Society (1999), the University of Waterloo 'Distinguished Teacher Award' (1999 and 2000), and the British Contact Lens Association's Dallos Award (2001). He has published over 50 papers and over 50 refereed abstracts, and has presented over 40 posters and 150 papers at conferences worldwide.

Debbie Jones is currently a Lecturer and Assistant Clinic Director in the School of Optometry at the University of Waterloo, Ontario, Canada. She graduated in Optometry in 1986 from City University in London, attained the Fellowship of the British College of Optometrists in 1992, completed her Diplomate in Contact Lens Practice in 1993, and became a Fellow of the American Academy of Optometry in 1995. Debbie has published 15 articles in optometric journals and presented over 10 posters at conferences in Europe and America. She is a recent co-recipient of one of the first Canada 'Foundation for Innovation' (CFI) grants.

Chapter 2: Microbial keratitis

Barry Weissman was educated at Santa Monica College, UCLA and the University of California at Berkeley (UCB), receiving a BSc in 1970. He received his OD (1972), MSc (1975), and PhD (1979) in Physiological Optics, all from the UCB School of Optometry. He has experience in private practice and was a member of the Contact Lens Service of the Hadassah-Hebrew University Medical School Department of Ophthalmology in Jerusalem, Israel, during 1975–76. He is currently a Professor of Ophthalmology and chief of the Contact Lens Service of the Jules Stein Eye Institute and Department of Ophthalmology, University of California Los Angeles (UCLA) School of Medicine in Los Angeles, California. Professor Weissman has received numerous prestigious awards, including the British Contact Lens Association (BCLA) Medal (2000), and the William Feinbloom (1996) and Max Schapero (1998) Awards of the American Academy of Optometry. He is a member of numerous professional and scientific bodies, and has authored approximately 150 research papers and textbook chapters, as well as four books in the field of contact lenses.

Bartly Mondino received his BA and then MD at Stanford University followed by an ophthalmology residency at Cornell University-New York Hospital. After completing a one-year fellowship in cornea-external disease at the University of Pittsburgh, Eye and Ear Hospital, he remained on the faculty there until his recruitment to the Jules Stein Eye Institute, UCLA School of Medicine, in 1982. Since January 1994 he has held the position of Chairman of the Department of Ophthalmology and Director of the Jules Stein Eye Institute. In October 1999 Dr Mondino was honoured as the recipient of the Bradley R. Straatsma Endowed Chair. In addition, he currently serves on the Board of Directors of the Charles R. Drew University of Medicine and Science and of the Braille Institute. Dr Mondino's research interests focus on ocular inflammation and immunity, and are detailed in over 200 publications. He has published extensively on autoimmune diseases of the external eye and contact lens-related corneal ulcers.

Chapter 3: Confocal microscopy

Nathan Efron completed his BScOptom (1977) and PhD (1983) at the University of Melbourne, Australia, and after two years of postdoctoral studies in Berkeley, USA, and Sydney, he returned to Melbourne as lecturer then senior lecturer responsible for contact lens education. In 1990 he took up the foundation Chair of Clinical Optometry at the University of Manchester Institute of Science and Technology (UMIST), in Manchester, UK, and established a contact lens research and consultancy unit known as *Eurolens Research*. He served as Head of Department from

1992 to 1997, and was admitted to the degree of Doctor of Science at UMIST in 1995. Professor Efron holds office in numerous professional bodies, and has served as President of both the Contact Lens Society of Australia (1981) and the British Contact Lens Association (BCLA) (1997). He lectures extensively worldwide, particularly in the field of the ocular response to contact lens wear, and has published over 400 scientific papers, abstracts, textbook chapters and books. Professor Efron has won a number of prestigious awards, including the *Optician* journal's 'Contribution to Optics' award (1997) and the BCLA Medal (2001).

Chapter 4: Light and electron microscopy

Jan P. G. Bergmanson received his optometric training and PhD at the City University, London. In addition, he obtained a Doctor of Optometry degree from Pennsylvania College of Optometry. Currently, he is Professor of Optometry at the University of Houston College of Optometry, where he is the founding Director of the Texas Eye Research and Technology Center. Professor Bergmanson has extensively researched and lectured internationally on subjects of corneal morphological response to contact lens wear, tear and ophthalmic solution effects on the ocular surface, histopathology of ocular tissues damaged by ultraviolet radiation, and the effects of the excimer laser on the cornea. In addition to private optometric practice, Professor Bergmanson – who is certified in Texas as a Therapeutic Optometrist and as an Optometric Glaucoma Specialist – has provided patient care in several hospital and university clinics. Professor Bergmanson is a Foundation Fellow of the College of Optometry (UK), a Fellow of the American Academy of Optometry (where he is a Diplomate in the Cornea and Contact Lens Section) and a member of the Texas Optometric Association, American Optometric Association, Association of Contact Lens Educators, and International Association of Contact Lens Educators. He is a council member of the International Society for Contact Lens Research and a lifetime honorary member of the Swedish and Dutch Optometric Associations, to which he also serves as a consultant. Professor Bergmanson was awarded the 1998 British Contact Lens Association Medal.

Chapter 5: Corneal topography

Stephen Klyce received his PhD in Physiology (vision research) from Yale University in 1971. Between 1972 and 1979 he based his professional research career in Ophthalmology at Stanford University. In 1979 Professor Klyce joined the faculty at the Louisiana State University (LSU) School of Medicine in New Orleans, where he conducts research in corneal physiology and biophysics. Currently he is a Professor of Ophthalmology and Anatomy/Cell Biology at LSU and Adjunct Professor of Biomedical Engineering at Tulane University. He has received numerous scientific honours including the 1990 Everett Kinsey Lecture (Contact Lens Association of Ophthalmologists), the 1991 Lans Distinguished Lecturer in Refractive Surgery (International Society for Refractive Surgery), the 1991 Max Schapero Memorial Lecture (American Academy of Optometry), the 1996 Whitney Sampson Lecture (American Academy of Ophthalmology), and the year 2000 Innovator's Award (American Society for Cataract and Refractive Surgery). He has served on the editorial boards of a number of scientific journals and is an active member of several professional societies including the Association for Research in Vision and Ophthalmology (Past President), the International Society for Eye Research (Past Councilor), and the International Society for Contact Lens Research (President). He has produced over 400 publications in the areas of corneal physiology, topography and refractive surgery.

1 Slit lamp biomicroscopy

Lyndon W. Jones and Deborah A. Jones

Introduction

The optical slit lamp biomicroscope[1] is a critically important instrument in contact lens practice, playing an essential role in the preliminary assessment and aftercare of the prospective and existing contact lens wearer. Indeed, it is extremely versatile for ophthalmic work generally; with the appropriate application of supplementary lenses and/or viewing techniques the instrument may be used to assess the condition of the vitreous, lens and retina from posterior pole to the ora serrata. In addition, various ancillary instruments will permit examination of the anterior chamber angle, measurement of intraocular pressure, corneal sensitivity and assessment of corneal thickness. Notwithstanding the importance of these various applications, this chapter will focus on the use of the slit lamp to examine the cornea, which is generally the pivotal procedure in a contact lens aftercare examination.

After describing the operation and clinical application of the slit lamp for examining the cornea of contact lens wearers, an overview of non-sight-threatening response of the cornea to contact lens wear will be presented. This overview will include consideration of changes that can be induced in all of the corneal layers and the limbus, the classical signs and symptoms, and an outline of the known or presumed aetiology and pathological processes involved. Appropriate treatment and management strategies will be detailed, along with comments on the likely prognosis for recovery of the various conditions. Advice on differential diagnosis will also be offered where appropriate.

Although sight-threatening ulcerative microbial keratitis is a condition that is also investigated using a slit lamp, this is a critical and sensitive aspect of contact lens practice supported by an extensive body of literature, and therefore deserves separate and detailed consideration.

[1]The optical slit lamp biomicroscope is variously referred to by the abbreviated term 'slit lamp' or 'biomicroscope'; for expediency, the term 'slit lamp' will be used throughout this book.

For this reason Chapter 2, by Weissman and Mondino, is devoted exclusively to this topic.

The slit lamp biomicroscope: principles and techniques

It is essential that the practitioner acquires a complete understanding of all of the features of the particular model of slit lamp biomicroscope that is to hand. A good starting point is to read the instruction manual from cover to cover (an exercise rarely undertaken in the fast pace of modern society) so that the location, suggested purpose and method of operation of every knob, dial, switch and filter is fully understood. This section will provide a general overview of the key features of the slit lamp and the various illumination and observation protocols that may be adopted.

The instrument

The instrument consists of a separate illumination system (the slit lamp) and viewing system (the biomicroscope), which have a common focal point and centre of rotation. A height control moves both systems simultaneously, and focusing and lateral movements are achieved via a joystick. This common control feature facilitates rapid and accurate positioning of the slit-beam on the area of interest and ensures that the microscope and illumination system are simultaneously in focus.

The illumination system

Virtually all slit lamp manufacturers have adopted the Koeller illumination system, which is optically almost identical to that of a 35 mm slide projector. A bright illumination system (producing approximately 600 000 lux) is a fundamental requirement for a slit lamp if subtle conditions are to be seen clearly. Whereas halogen or xenon lamps are more expensive than tungsten lamps, they are the preferred illumination source because they provide a brighter light, last longer, have better colour rendering and generate less heat. Illumination brightness is controlled by a rheostat or multiposition switch, such that brightness can be adjusted to obtain the correct balance between patient comfort and optimal visibility of the area of interest.

   The slit within the illumination system must have sharply demarcated edges. The slit width and height must be easily adjustable such that a patch of any shape – from a slit to a circle – may be projected; this will increase the variety of illumination methods possible. A graduated slit width is particularly useful when measuring the size of a lesion. An ability to rotate the lamp housing such that the slit may be used in meridians away from the vertical is useful, particularly if a protractor scale is included. Such a system enables, for example, the angle of rotation of a soft toric lens away from the vertical to be accurately measured. The slit beam must also have the facility to be displaced or offset sideways ('decoupled'). This ability to break the linkage between the illumination and observation systems facilitates indirect illumination techniques.

A number of filters are incorporated into the illumination system, and these are used to enhance the visibility of certain conditions:

- Green ('red-free') filter – enhances contrast when looking for corneal and iris vascularization, since red vessels appear black if viewed through such a filter. In addition, this filter may be used to increase the visibility of rose bengal staining on both the cornea and conjunctiva.
- Neutral density (ND) filter – reduces beam brightness and increases comfort for the patient.
- Polarizing filter – reduces unwanted specular reflections and can be useful for enhancing the visibility of subtle defects.
- Diffusing filter – diffuses the illumination source over a wide area and is used to provide broad, unfocused illumination for low-magnification viewing of the general ocular surface.
- Cobalt blue filter – provides a suitable means of exciting sodium fluorescein for examination of ocular surface integrity. Illumination of fluorescein with cobalt blue light of 460–490 nm produces a greenish light of maximum emission 520 nm. Any abraded area will absorb fluorescein and display a fluorescent green area against a general blue background (Figure 1.1). The filter is occasionally used on its own to aid in the diagnosis of keratoconus. A frequent finding in this corneal ectasia is Fleischer's ring, which is formed by annular iron deposition within the stroma at the base of the cone. The iron pigment is often difficult to see in white light but will usually appear in greater contrast when viewed through the cobalt blue filter.
- Kodak Wratten #12 (yellow) filter – this is not a filter contained within the illumination system but a barrier filter that must be placed in front of the viewing system. It significantly enhances the contrast of any fluorescent staining observed with the cobalt blue filter as it allows transmission of the green, fluorescent light but blocks the blue light reflected from the corneal surface (Courtney

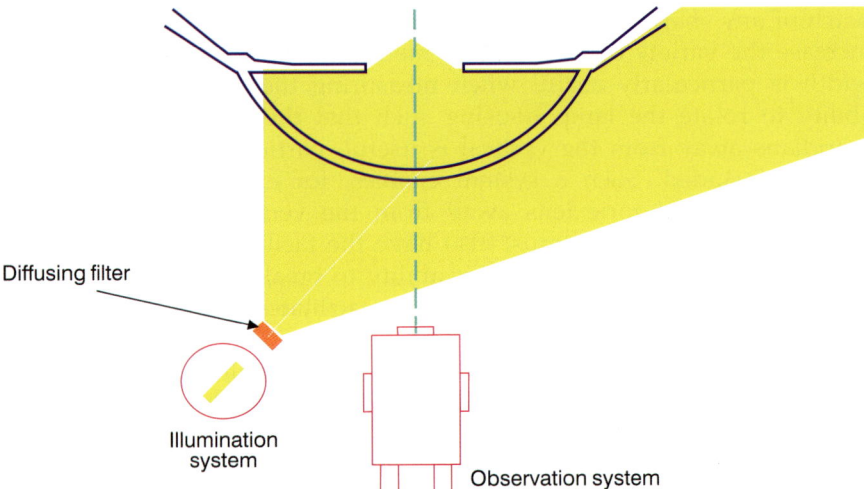

Diffusing filter

Illumination system

Observation system

Figure 1.1 Diagrammatic representation of diffuse illumination (Adapted from Zantos and Cox, 1994)

and Lee, 1982; Back, 1988). This filter improves the contrast and facilitates the detection of subtle forms of staining that may not be visible without the filter. Custom-made barrier filters for certain slit lamps are available from the manufacturers. Inexpensive hand-held versions may be constructed by using a cardboard mask and Lee filters #101 Yellow, which can be purchased from a variety of suppliers. In addition, the interposition of an excitation filter in the illumination system (such as a Wratten #47 or Ealing #35–5297) will produce even better results (Cox and Fonn, 1991).

The microscope

In addition to the illumination system described above, the slit lamp requires a viewing system to provide a clear image of the eye, which has sufficient magnification for the practitioner to view all structures of interest. Magnification is an important issue and the slit lamp should be capable of providing magnifications of up to 40×, which may be achieved through interchangeable eyepieces and/or variable magnification of the slit lamp objective (Henson, 1996). Magnification greater than 40× in an optical viewing instrument is counterproductive as small involuntary eye movements will render the image too unstable to view. Much higher magnification (680×) is possible with the confocal microscope, as will be described by Efron *et al.* in Chapter 3.

Ideally the practitioner should be able to change magnification swiftly and easily, and greater utility will be afforded to those slit lamps that have three or more objectives to choose from. Zoom systems have the added advantage of allowing the practitioner to focus on a particular structure without losing sight of it during changes in magnification. The magnified image must also be clear, and it is important to choose a slit lamp with a high-quality optical system. The microscope should also have excellent resolution and a good depth of field; however, these factors are inversely linked and so a compromise must be accepted.

Illumination and observation techniques

Mastering the available illumination techniques possible with the slit lamp is essential if the instrument is to be used to its full potential; practice with the instrument is critical to becoming comfortable with its subtle but extensive variety of uses. In reality it is impractical to completely dissociate the viewing techniques as in one field of view several different methods of illumination simultaneously present themselves. The experienced observer is then able to assimilate useful information without necessarily having to resort to differing physical adjustments of the slit lamp. The optical effects produced by the incident beam of light depend upon the tissues illuminated and their transparency, as reflection, scattering or absorption can all occur to various degrees.

Diffuse illumination

A ground-glass filter is placed in the focused light beam of the slit lamp. This defocuses and diffuses the light to give a broad, even illumination over the entire field of view and is generally used to provide low-magnification views of the anterior segment (Figures 1.1 and 1.2). Typical uses include viewing soft contact lens fitting characteristics, contact lens deposits, external eyelid anomalies and general conjunctival appearance.

Direct focal illumination

This describes any illumination technique where the slit beam and viewing system are focused coincidentally. The illumination beam is turned up as brightly as possible (ensuring that the patient remains comfortable) and placed at a separation of 40–60° on the side of the microscope corresponding to the section of the cornea to be viewed. The

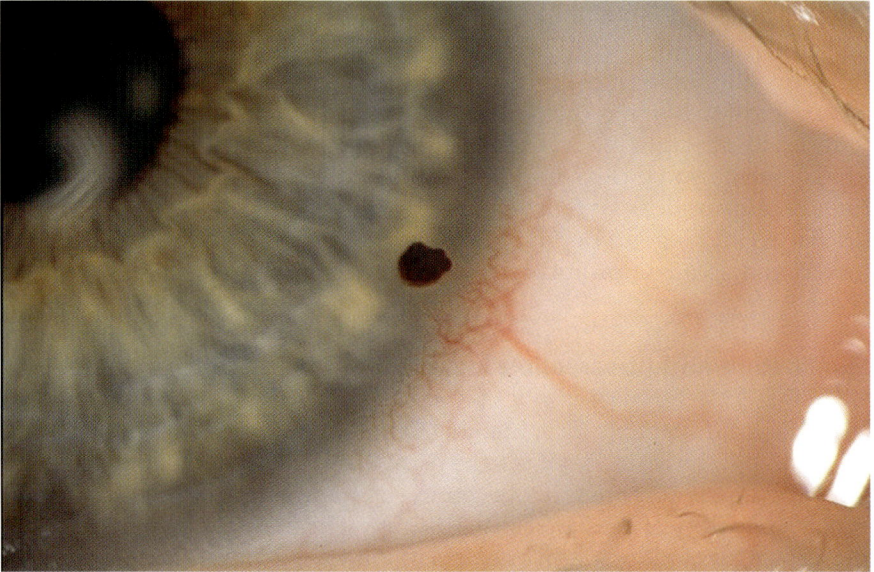

Figure 1.2 Diffuse illumination view of an embedded metallic foreign body in the cornea. Note how the depth of the foreign body cannot be determined using this technique

beam is swept smoothly across the ocular surface and the illumination system moved across to the opposite side as the beam crosses the midpoint of the cornea. Typically a beam width of 2–3 mm is chosen initially, and this may be reduced so as to bring more contrast (due to less light scatter) to an area of interest. While scanning the external ocular surface, a low–medium magnification is initially chosen and the magnification is increased if a particular area needs to be examined more closely.

Parallelepiped

Using the setup described above, a 0.5–2.0 mm wide illuminating beam is scanned over the ocular surface (Figure 1.3). This permits assessment of the location, width and height of any object within the cornea or adjacent structures (Figure 1.4). The parallelepiped is the most commonly used direct illumination technique and is employed, for example, to assess corneal scarring, infiltrates and corneal staining.

Optic section

Once an area or object of interest is located the beam width is narrowed to approximately 0.2 mm to 'cross-section' the corneal tissue. This

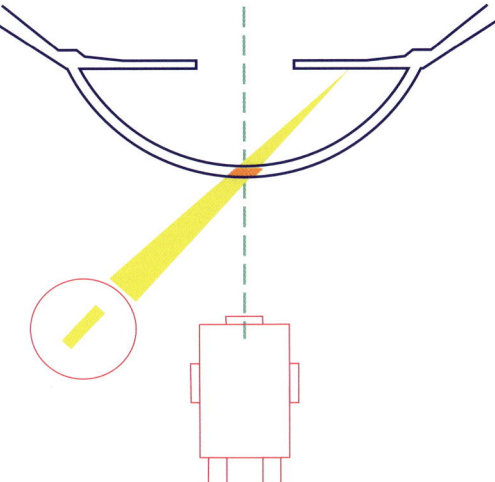

Figure 1.3 Diagrammatic representation of a parallelepiped (Adapted from Zantos and Cox, 1994)

provides the ability to accurately assess the depth of an object within the corneal layers (Figure 1.5). Typical uses include assessment of the depth of a foreign body, location of a corneal scar (Figure 1.6) and determining whether tissue within an area of staining is excavated, flat or raised.

Oblique illumination

This is infrequently used in contact lens practice, but is nonetheless a useful technique. Oblique illumination is achieved by setting up a parallelepiped and then moving the illumination system away from the

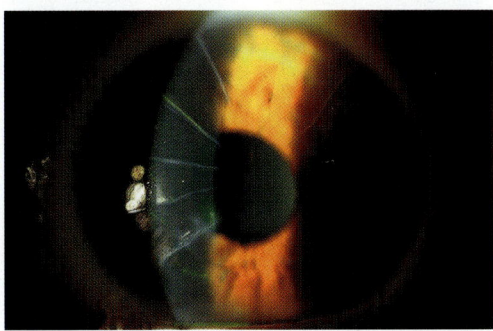

Figure 1.4 Parallelepiped view of radial keratotomy scars. Note how the depth of the incisions cannot be determined using this technique. Also note how the scars are not visible to the right of the direct beam in the light reflected from the iris (Courtesy of Rosaline Robinson)

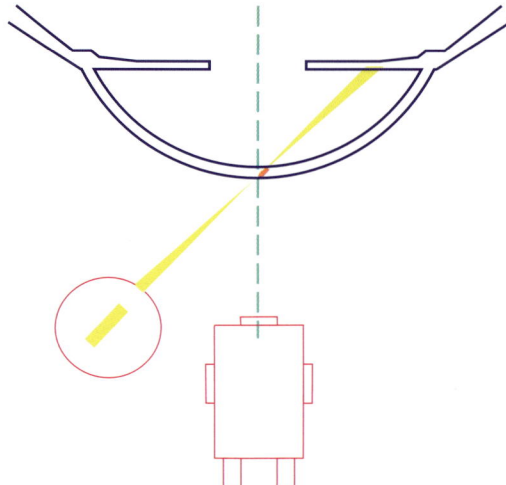

Figure 1.5 Diagrammatic representation of an optic section (Adapted from Zantos and Cox, 1994)

observation system until the angle between them is close to 90°. The illumination arm is adjusted until the light beam is almost tangential to the object of interest. Any raised areas cast a shadow, and this technique is particularly useful for viewing subtle defects within the iris architecture and subtle changes to the epithelial surface.

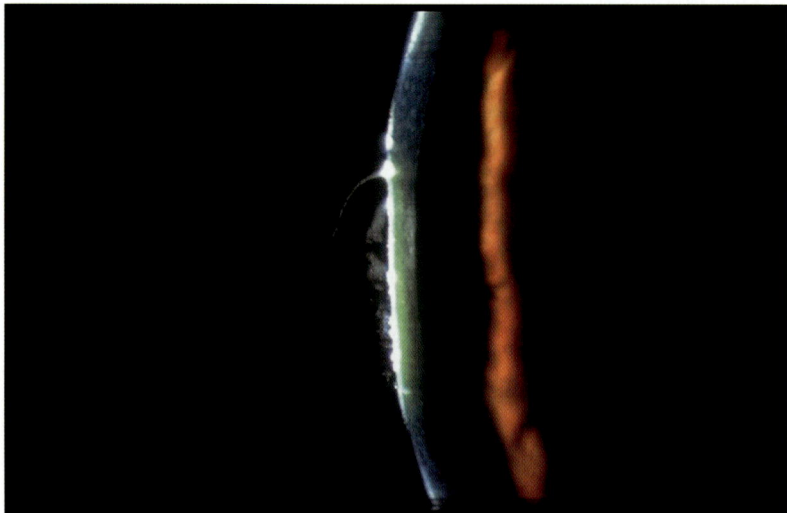

Figure 1.6 Optic section of a corneal scar. Note how the use of this technique clearly enables the location of the scar to be determined and how the cornea is thinned centrally (Courtesy of Desmond Fonn)

Specular reflection

This is a specific case of a parallelepiped setup, where the angle of the incident slit beam is equal to the angle of the observation axis through one of the oculars. At this angle (typically 40–50°) the illumination beam is reflected from the smooth surfaces of the anterior segment and provides a mirror-like reflection (Figure 1.7). Such specular images occur

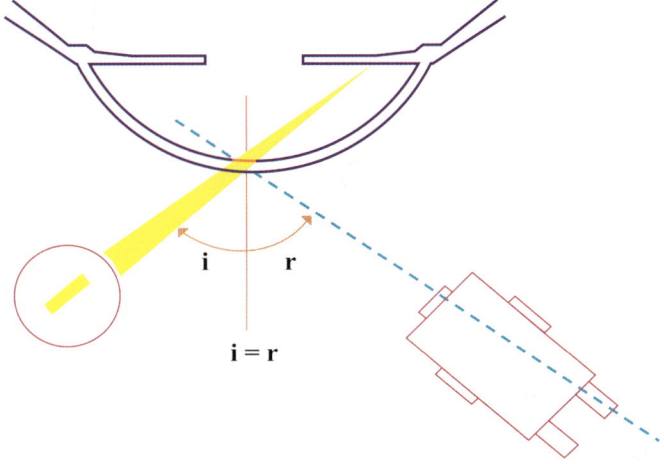

Figure 1.7 Diagrammatic representation of specular reflection (Adapted from Zantos and Cox, 1994)

at every interface between structures of different refractive indexes. The technique of specular reflection is typically used to view the endothelium (Figure 1.8), tear film quality, 'orange-peel' appearance of the anterior lens surface, and front surface wetting of a contact lens. Even at 40× magnification only a gross clinical judgement of the endothelium can be made as individual cells are barely visible.

Indirect illumination

This refers to any technique where the focus of the illuminating beam does not coincide with the focal point of the observation system. Indirect illumination can be achieved by 'uncoupling' the instrument and manually displacing the slit beam to the side. However, it is possible to effect indirect illumination without uncoupling the instrument; this is achieved by directing a slit beam onto a section of the cornea adjacent to that of interest, and to direct gaze to the side of the directly illuminated section.

The following two specific types of indirect illumination are possible.

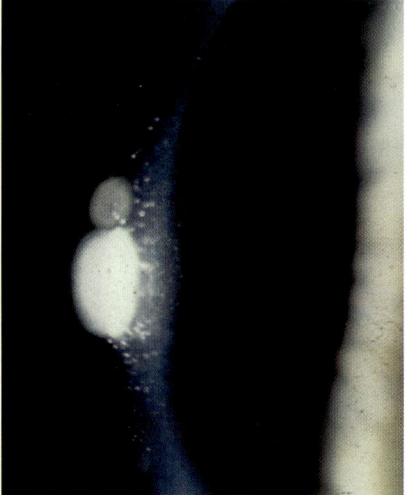

Figure 1.8 Specular reflection view of endothelial guttae, which are clearly visible to the right of the specular reflex

Sclerotic scatter

This technique is used to investigate any subtle changes in corneal clarity occurring over a large area, such as central corneal oedema. The slit lamp is set up for a wide-angle parallelepiped (45–60°) and the viewing system is focused centrally. The beam is manually offset ('uncoupled') and focused on the limbus. The slit beam is totally internally reflected across

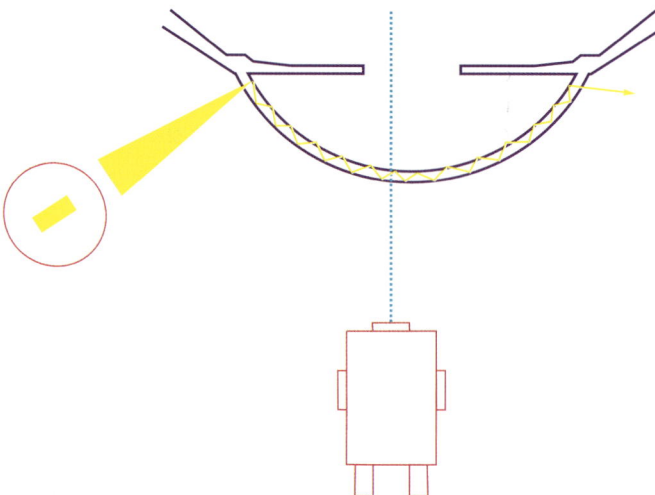

Figure 1.9 Diagrammatic representation of sclerotic scatter (Adapted from Zantos and Cox, 1994)

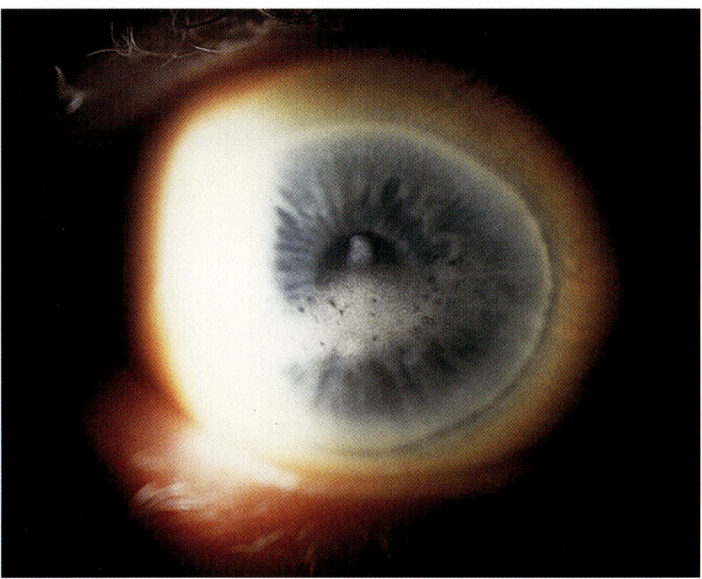

Figure 1.10 Band keratopathy made visible by the use of sclerotic scatter. The area over which the keratopathy extends is clearly seen using this technique

the cornea and a bright limbal glow is seen around the entire cornea (Figure 1.9). Any specific area of abnormality, such as a corneal scar, will interrupt the beam in its passage and produce a light reflection in the otherwise dark cornea (Figure 1.10).

Retro-illumination

This refers to any technique in which light is reflected from the iris, anterior lens surface or retina, and is used to back-illuminate an area more anteriorly positioned (Figure 1.11). The area may be seen against a light background (direct retro-illumination) or a dark background (indirect retro-illumination), depending whether or not the illumination and viewing systems are coincident. Direct retro-illumination is used most often, whereby corneal opacities will appear black against a bright field. This technique is particularly useful for examining epithelial microcysts, neovascularization, scars, degenerations and dystrophies (Figure 1.12).

The slit lamp routine

As with all aspects of ocular examination, practitioners should develop a routine procedure that enables coverage of all aspects of the assessment in a logical, systematic and consistent manner. The slit lamp examination of

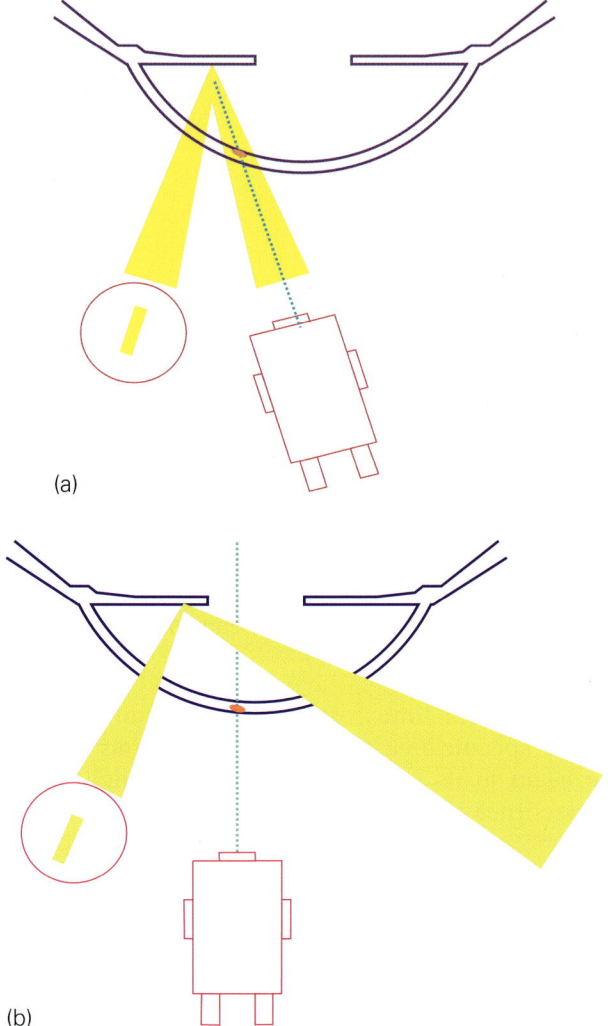

(a)

(b)

Figure 1.11 Diagrammatic representation of direct (a) and indirect (b) retro-illumination (Adapted from Zantos and Cox, 1994)

the eye requires deployment of several different illumination techniques. The ability to detect and diagnose anterior segment conditions often depends upon the skill of the observer to select and correctly apply the appropriate technique. The sequence of the examination will vary from one practitioner to another. Usually, the examination will start with low magnification and diffuse illumination for general observation, with the magnification increasing and more specific illumination techniques being

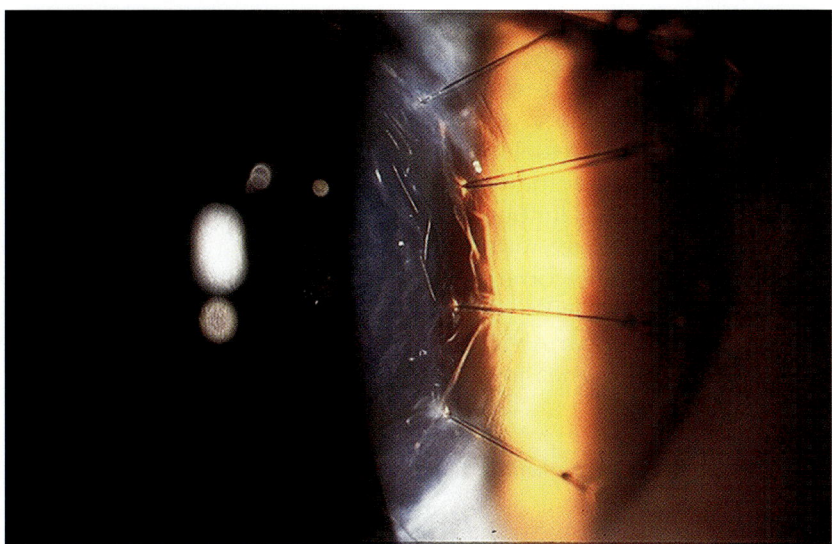

Figure 1.12 View of sutures in a patient following penetrating keratoplasty. Note how the sutures and corneal wrinkling are seen in indirect illumination via light reflected from the iris

employed to view structures in more detail as the examination progresses.

A typical routine is outlined below. With practice and experience, practitioners will inevitably develop their own approach.

Overall view: low magnification with wide diffuse beam

The examination should begin with a number of sweeps across the anterior segment and adnexa, while using a broad diffused beam and low magnification. The lid margins and lashes should be examined for signs of marginal blepharitis or hordeolum, and the patency of the meibomian glands assessed by gently squeezing the lids. The bulbar conjunctiva is then assessed for hyperaemia and for the presence of any abnormalities such as pinguecula or pterygia. The superior and inferior palpebral conjunctivae are examined to check for hyperaemia, follicles and papillae.

Corneal and limbal examination: medium magnification with 2 mm wide beam

The diffusing filter is removed and the corneal examination begins by uncoupling the slit lamp illumination and observation systems and examining the cornea for gross opacification using the sclerotic scatter illumination technique. The slit lamp is then recoupled and a series of observation sweeps is carried out across the cornea. The limbal vasculature is examined to assess the degree of physiological corneal vascularization (blood vessels overlying clear cornea), differentiating this from neovascularization (new blood vessels growing into clear cornea). Blood vessels at the limbus are best observed using both direct illumination and indirect retro-illumination, looking to the side of the illuminated area of the cornea. Once the limbus has been assessed the cornea is examined with a parallelepiped to look for any gross abnormalities, before narrowing the beam and increasing the magnification to examine the cornea in greater detail.

Corneal examination: high magnification with narrow beam

An optic section is established and, with high magnification, the slit lamp is systematically swept from side to side across the cornea to look for features of particular interest. At this point a number of illumination techniques can simultaneously be used. In addition to using direct illumination to look for any subtle opacification, stromal striae, or folds in the posterior limiting lamina (Descemet's membrane), retro-illumination is used to detect the presence of microcysts, and specular reflection is employed to inspect the endothelium and tear film.

Staining examination

It is essential that the cornea be examined with various stains during contact lens aftercare checks and in cases where patients complain of dry eyes; no contact lens aftercare should be considered complete without a staining examination taking place. Sodium fluorescein is a vital stain. It reveals the presence of damaged epithelial tissue and is the best means of judging corneal integrity. Rose bengal is an iodine derivative of fluorescein that binds to mucus and cellular components. It is useful in the diagnosis of dry eye, in which it is seen binding to degenerate cells on the corneal surface. Lissamine green is a relatively new vital stain which has a similar action to rose bengal but does not sting on instillation.

Recording of clinical observations

Equally important to carrying out the examination is the recording of the results obtained. In law, if an action is not recorded it is not deemed to have taken place and practitioners must attempt to record and quantify what observations have been made. It is vitally important to ensure that such measurements are reproducible and repeatable if they are to be used successfully. Practitioners constantly record slit lamp observations in order to make clinical decisions. Descriptive terms such as 'acceptable', 'slight', 'bumpy' or 'smooth' are too subjective in nature and are likely to result in variations in interpretation both over time and between practitioners. A suitable system or systems must be used if the change in such clinical observations is to be accurately monitored.

One option is to physically measure the size of the object of interest. For example, blood vessel infiltration into the cornea can be directly recorded by using a graduated graticule placed within the objective eyepiece. Some slit lamp manufacturers produce custom-made graticule eyepieces, but these are often expensive. An alternative suggestion involves converting the spare eyepieces often provided with slit lamps into dedicated graticule eyepieces, which are subsequently used when a measurement is required. These spare eyepieces can be converted relatively inexpensively by obtaining graticules from a variety of sources, including those listed in Table 1.1.

Table 1.1 Sources of eyepiece graticules

Company	Address	Telephone	Fax	Email
Pyser (SGI) Ltd (Graticules Division)	Fircroft way, Edenbridge, Kent TN8 6HA, UK	01732 864111	01732 865544	sales@pyser.sgi.com
Electron Microscopy Sciences	PO Box 251, 321 Morris Road, Fort Washington, Pa 19034, USA	215 646 1566	215 646 8931	sgkcck@aol.com

Certain objects may be counted. For example, the progression of stromal striae or epithelial microcysts may be monitored by physically counting them. However, the majority of slit lamp observations can be neither counted nor measured. The most reliable recording technique for use with features that cannot be measured depends upon the practitioner assigning grading scales to their clinical observations (Woods, 1989). Each observation may be regarded as part of a continuous scale, which is assigned a grade based on the clinical observation. This grade serves as a standard by which any future observation can be judged. One frequently used option is the continuous five-point scale (Woods, 1989), such as that in Table 1.2.

More sensitive results are found if the scale is expanded to cover a range from 0 to 10 (Bailey *et al.*, 1991; Lloyd, 1992). One possible adaptation, as described by Lloyd (1992), is to use plus or minus increments (e.g. 0, 1−, 1, 1+, etc.), which would change the scale in Table 1.2 from a five-point scale to a nine-point scale. This scale may be

Table 1.2 Severity grading scale

Numerical	Descriptive	Meaning
Grade 0	Normal	No action
Grade 1	Slight	Not clinically significant
Grade 2	Moderate	May require intervention
Grade 3	Severe	Requires intervention
Grade 4	Very severe	Requires medical intervention

modified to include all the major clinical findings observed during a slit lamp examination. Several grading systems have been published (Mandell, 1987; Zantos and Cox, 1994) but practitioners can easily devise their own. Recently the subject of grading has received considerable interest due to the release of grading systems based on photographs (CCLRU, 1997) or artist-rendered paintings (Figure 1.13; Efron, 1999, 2000; Efron *et al.*, 2001)).

Photography and video recording

Photography of the eye is a comprehensive means of recording clinical findings. A 35 mm camera can either be incorporated into the slit lamp optics as a designed feature or by attaching the camera in place of one of the eyepieces of the microscope system. An alternative to still photography is to add a video attachment. The availability of miniature video cameras makes this a highly practical option. In addition to providing an instant image, which may be of value to demonstrate specific points to the patient, the still or movie video camera may also be adapted to aid measurement for research purposes. Still and movie digital cameras can also be used to record slit lamp images. The most versatile arrangement is to interface a slit lamp-mounted digital camera – which is capable of capturing both still and movie images – with a computer that has image

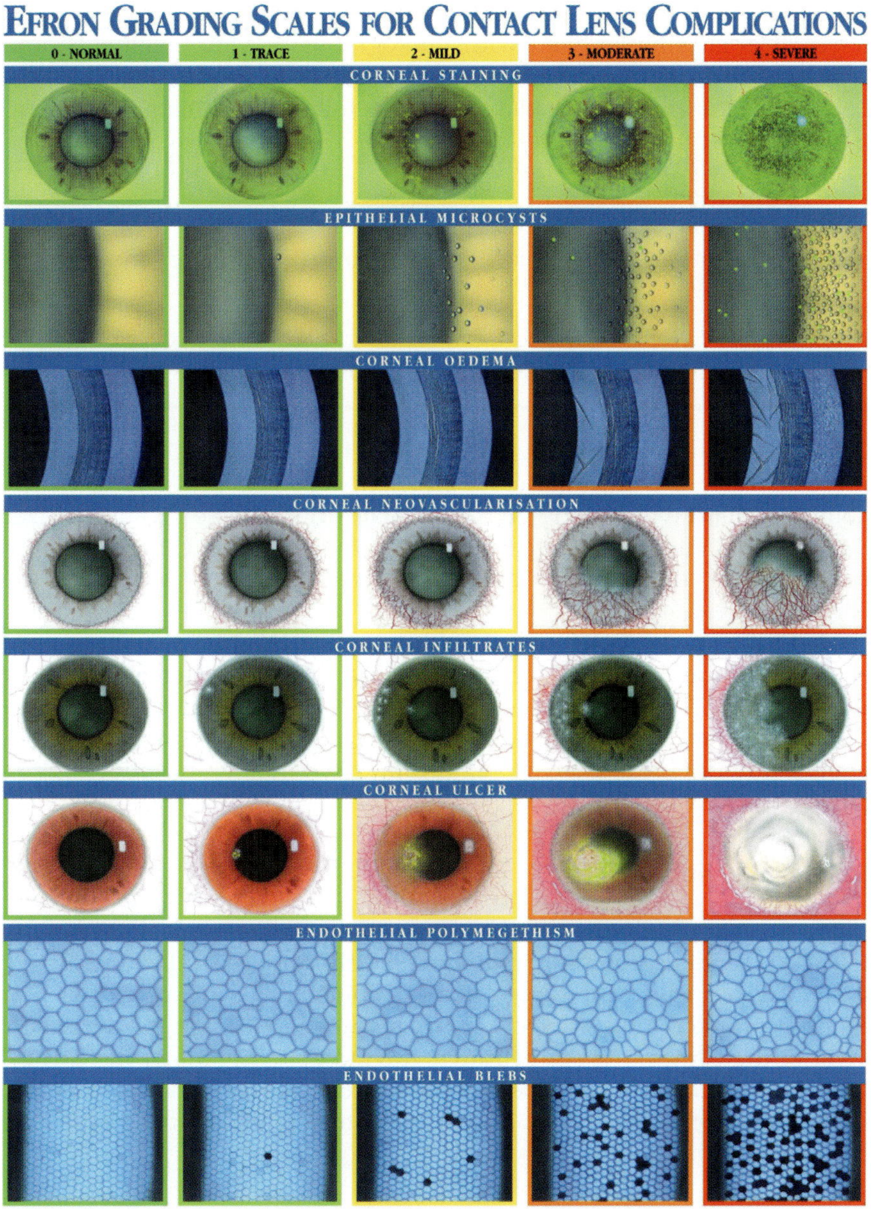

Figure 1.13 Efron grading scales for corneal complications of contact lens wear. An A4-sized plastic-encapsulated version of these grading scales in presentation slip-case can be obtained without charge from Biocompatibles-Hydron (e-mail: gradingscales@biocompatibles.co.uk)

storage/manipulation software. This arrangement has significant advantages in that the image is obtained immediately, image storage and
retrieval is far simpler than with photographs or video-segments, and
comparisons from one visit to the next are easy to conduct.

Further information is available from the following sources concerning:

- photography – see Cox and Fonn, 1991; Lowe, 1991; Phelps-Brown,
  1991; Bowen, 1993;
- videography – see Hammack, 1995;
- digital imaging – see Cox, 1995; Krasnow, 1997; Meyler and Burnett-
  Hodd, 1998.

Effects of contact lenses on the cornea

Contact lenses have a wide variety of effects on all layers of the cornea,
most of which are attributable to either their mechanical effect or their
ability to retard oxygen flow to the corneal surface. Table 1.3 summarizes
the principal effects of contact lenses on the cornea and, for simplicity,
divides these complications by way of the various layers/areas of the
cornea affected.

This section will briefly deal with some of the more common and
significant complications that practitioners are likely to encounter in their
daily practice. More details on the aetiology and management of these
conditions can be found in texts dealing specifically with contact lens
complications (Tomlinson, 1992; Efron, 1999; Jones and Jones, 2000;
Silbert, 2000).

Epithelial changes

There is a very high rate of metabolic activity in the corneal epithelium
that is dependent upon a continuous supply of oxygen. It is necessary,
therefore, to consider the clinical signs of epithelial oxygen deprivation so
that this problem can be detected early and rectified. Being the outermost
layer of the cornea, the epithelium is the most susceptible of the corneal
layers to mechanical insult as a result of contact lens wear, so it is also
important that clinicians are aware of strategies for detecting epithelial
damage and managing the potential consequences.

Hypoxia

Since the epithelium derives virtually all its oxygen supply from the
atmosphere, contact lenses have the capability to interrupt that supply. In
this regard, rigid lenses have an advantage over hydrogel lenses because

Table 1.3 Summary of common complications induced by contact lenses	
Layer/area of the cornea	*Complication*
Epithelium	Hypoxia Microcysts Vacuoles Corneal staining 'Smile' (desiccation/dehydration) Hypersensitivity/toxicity '3&9' staining Mechanical
Stroma	Hypoxia Striae Folds Inflammation Infiltrative keratitis (IK) Contact lens peripheral ulcer (CLPU) Contact lens-related acute red eye (CLARE) Adenoviral
Endothelium	Hypoxia Polymegethism Blebs
Limbus	Hypoxia Limbal hyperaemia Vascularization Staining Superior limbic keratoconjunctivitis secondary to contact lens wear (CL-SLK) Superior epithelial arcuate lesions (SEAL)

(1) they do not cover all of the cornea, and (2) they support an exchange of tears that serves to reoxygenate the tear film beneath the lens. Soft lenses rely upon gas transmission through the lens, with the ultimate material capable of facilitating this process being silicone hydrogels (Sweeney, 2000). The two main clinical signs of epithelial hypoxia are microcysts and vacuoles.

Microcysts

Epithelial microcysts are 15–50 μm diameter epithelial vesicles that are observed in the superficial epithelium, typically 2–3 months after commencing extended wear (Zantos, 1983; Holden and Sweeney, 1991). Small numbers are observed in 10–20% of those wearing lenses on a daily-wear basis, and increased numbers are seen in patients wearing extended-wear lenses, which have a low oxygen permeability. They occur due to hypoxia and are believed to consist of necrotic cellular tissue or cellular debris and arise due to an alteration of the mitotic state of the basal epithelial cells. Patients are typically asymptomatic and the presence of microcysts acts as a useful indicator of the degree of hypoxic stress experienced by the cornea. They are viewed using marginal retro-illumination (Figure 1.14) and display a characteristic reversed illumination due to their refractive index being higher than the surrounding tissue (Zantos, 1983). Microcysts form in the deepest layers

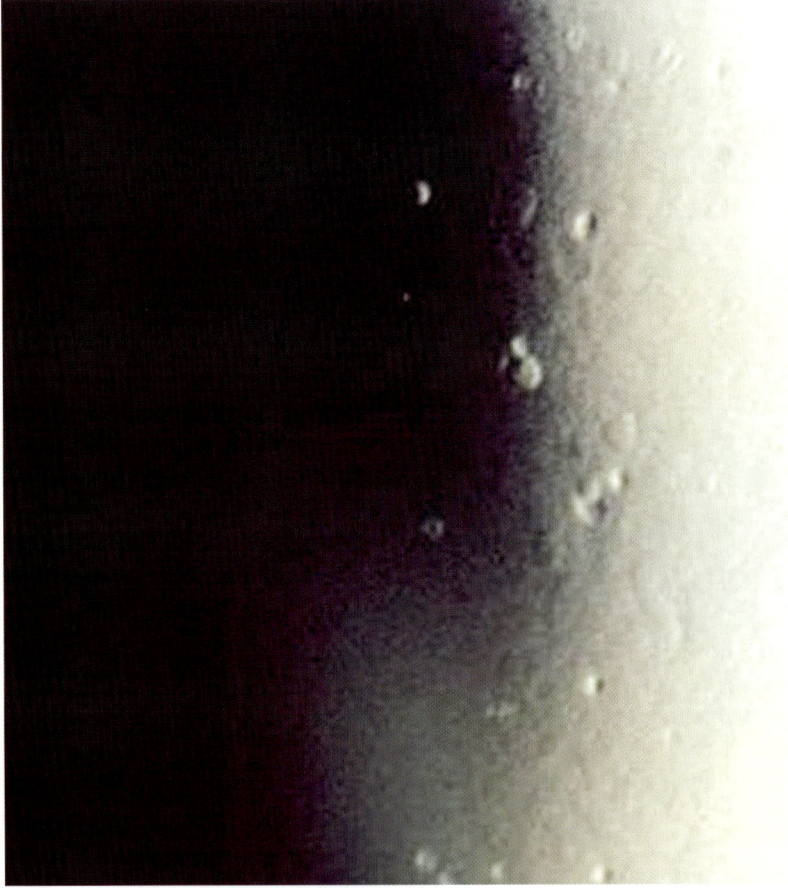

Figure 1.14 Epithelial microcysts, displaying characteristic reversed illumination due to their high refractive index (Courtesy of Steve Zantos)

of the epithelium and gradually move forwards to the epithelial surface, where they may stain as they break through the epithelial surface, resulting in a central superficial punctate keratitis. Following cessation of lens wear or a change from extended to daily wear the number of microcysts initially increases and then resolves as the corneal metabolic activity returns to normal levels (Holden and Sweeney, 1991). Preliminary results with high *Dk* silicone hydrogel materials indicate that the enhanced oxygen transmissibility obtained with such materials largely eliminates the microcystic response (MacDonald *et al.*, 1995; Keay *et al.*, 2000).

Vacuoles
Epithelial vacuoles also occur in response to chronic hypoxia. These fluid-filled bubbles or cysts in the epithelium are almost perfectly round, are usually few in number and are easily distinguished from microcysts in that they show unreversed illumination, confirming that they have a lower refractive index than the surrounding tissue (Zantos, 1983).

Corneal staining

As described above, epithelial integrity is assessed with the slit lamp using sodium fluorescein and a cobalt blue filter. Uptake of fluorescein by the epithelium occurs when cell membrane permeability is increased, cell junctions are damaged or epithelial cell loss occurs (Back, 1988). Fluorescein also pools in areas where there is a depression in the corneal surface, such as that which occurs in the presence of corneal dimple-veil staining (Jones and Jones, 1995). Many non-contact lens wearers also exhibit ocular staining, particularly in cases of active disease such as dry eye, keratitis and conjunctivitis. Estimates of the prevalence of corneal staining indicates that 50–70% of patients exhibit some degree of corneal staining and that contact lens wearers exhibit greater levels of staining than non-wearers (Josephson and Caffery, 1992; Guillon *et al.*, 1995; Begley *et al.*, 1996; Schwallie *et al.*, 1997; Jalbert *et al.*, 1999). However, such staining is often clinically insignificant and the percentage of subjects in which clinically significant staining occurs is probably closer to 15% (Guillon *et al.*, 1995). The degree of staining is similar in daily wear and extended wear of hydrogel lenses (Jalbert *et al.*, 1999) and is variable across time and between subjects (Schwallie *et al.*, 1997). The intensity of staining increases with multiple sequential instillations of fluorescein and longer viewing times (Korb and Herman, 1979). The central cornea stains less than peripheral areas and most staining occurs in the inferior quadrant of the cornea (Begley *et al.*, 1996; Schwallie *et al.*, 1997; Jalbert *et al.*, 1999).

Once recorded, the cause of the staining must be ascertained and appropriate action taken to remedy the situation, where necessary. It is important to decide what level of corneal staining is unacceptable and hence necessitates a period without lens wear; however, a well established criterion does not exist. Back (1988) suggests that lens removal is indicated when diffusion of fluorescein occurs within 60 seconds and/ or widespread punctate or moderate areas of coalescing stain are seen. In such circumstances the lenses should be removed for approximately 24 hours in cases of slight diffusion, 48–72 hours with moderate diffusion, and at least seven days in cases of immediate, widespread diffusion.

The following specific types of corneal staining require elaboration as to their aetiology and management.

'Smile' staining

Slit lamp examination of soft lens-wearing patients will often reveal a coarse inferior punctate staining of an arcuate fashion extending from 4 to 8 o'clock in the lower third of the cornea, 2–3 mm in from the limbus (Figure 1.15). These coarse punctate dots stain with fluorescein and rose

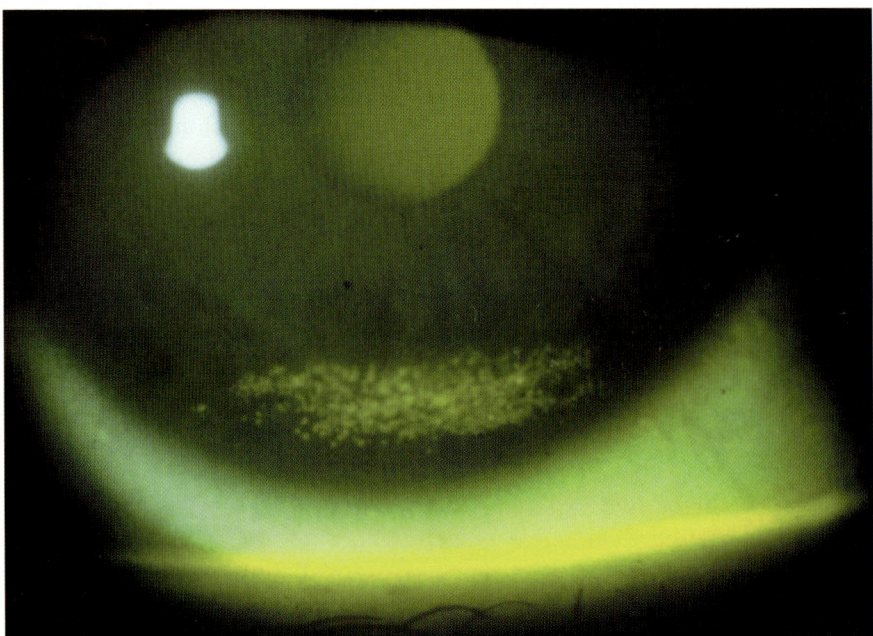

Figure 1.15 Dehydration-induced inferior 'smile' stain following the use of a thin, mid-water content disposable lens in a patient with a partial blink reflex

bengal, but may be visible in white light as small, white, 'snowflake-like' opacities. This staining is generally referred to as inferior arcuate staining (Zadnik and Mutti, 1985) or 'smile stain'. Corneal staining with a similar appearance may also occur centrally, particularly with ultra-thin high-water-content lenses (McNally *et al.*, 1986), where it occurs in almost all cases after as little as two hours of wear. While smile defects are typically superficial, central staining with thin high-water-content lenses often indicates a full epithelial thickness defect that can extend into the stroma.

The mechanism behind the formation of these two types of staining is probably similar, occurring through initial lens dehydration (Orsborn and Zantos, 1988), depletion of the post-lens tear film (Little and Bruce, 1994) and subsequent staining through epithelial desiccation. Contact lens dehydration and corneal staining remain intimately linked, being related in part to lens design, polymer type and environmental factors. Increased dehydration and corneal staining is typically found with high-water-content ionic lenses, thinner lenses (being related to both lens design and back vertex power) and in low-humidity environments (Orsborn and Zantos, 1988; Helton and Watson, 1991; Grimmer, 1992). Significant inter-subject differences are also commonly found (Brennan *et al.*, 1988) and may be explained by variations in lens power, palpebral aperture size, epithelial fragility, post-lens tear film thickness, blinking frequency and tear pH/osmolarity (Efron *et al.*, 1987).

A specific causative factor in the production of 'smile' staining is that of incomplete blinking, resulting in local lens dehydration (Collins *et al.*, 1989). Smile staining is a common finding among soft lens wearers who have an incomplete blink reflex, and may also be seen in non-lens wearers who exhibit an incomplete blink pattern (Abelson and Holly, 1977). If the staining is minor no treatment is usually required and subjects simply require careful follow-up. Remedial treatment for symptomatic subjects or those with clinically significant staining includes regular use of ocular lubricants, blinking exercises, locally placed humidifiers and switching to either low-water-content lenses (Orsborn and Zantos, 1988) or thicker higher-water-content lenses (Zadnik and Mutti, 1985). Lubricants alone are often inadequate in severe staining (Collins *et al.*, 1989). Whereas lubricants may alleviate feelings of dryness they do not affect the level of dehydration (Efron *et al.*, 1991) and are unlikely to significantly influence the degree of corneal staining.

Solution hypersensitivity/toxicity staining
A small percentage of contact lens wearers may exhibit a toxic or hypersensitivity reaction upon exposure to various elements within a care regimen, in particular thimerosal, chlorhexidine or benzalkonium chloride (Mondino *et al.*, 1982; Atkins and Allsopp, 1996). A more acute

reaction may also be seen in patients who inadvertently insert their lenses directly from hydrogen peroxide, without neutralization taking place, and in subjects using certain enzyme removal systems. Patients are often asymptomatic, but may complain of reduced wearing time, dryness and stinging on lens insertion. The classic slit lamp signs include diffuse punctate staining of the superficial corneal epithelium (Figure 1.16),

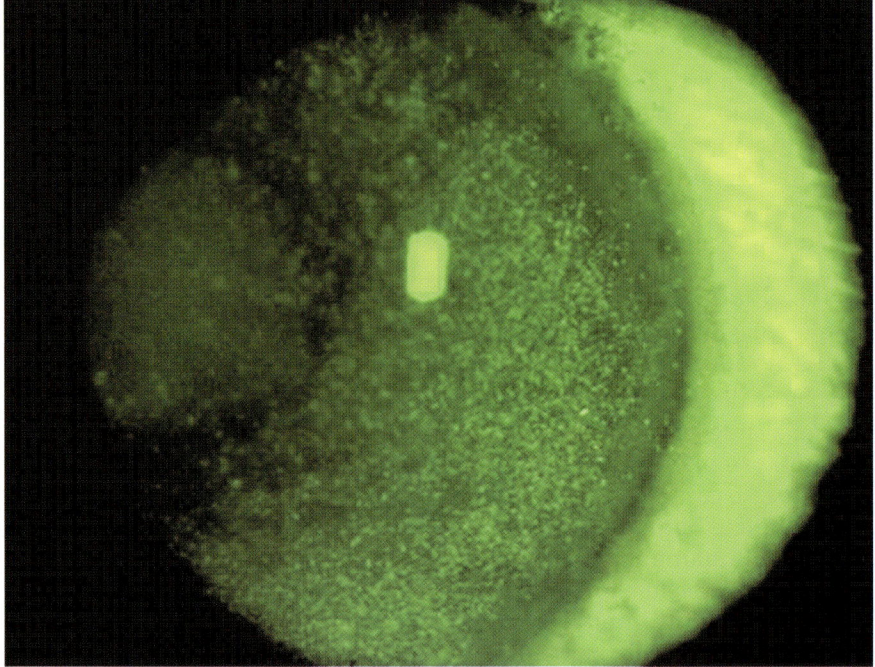

Figure 1.16 Diffuse punctate epithelial staining due to a hypersensitivity reaction to a contact lens care system (Courtesy of Ian Cox)

generalized conjunctival hyperaemia, and increased hyperaemia of the palpebral conjunctiva (Dougal, 1992; Caffery and Josephson, 2000; Davis and Lebow, 2000). Initial management in all such cases includes replacement of existing lenses or long-term soaking of the lenses in saline to purge out the causative agent. In minor cases, simply switching to an unpreserved system such as one based on hydrogen peroxide or switching to a system that uses a different preservative is often sufficient to alleviate both symptoms and signs. In more severe conditions, a 1–2 day period of cessation of lens wear is indicated, particularly in cases caused by insufficiently neutralized lenses previously soaked in peroxide. Most cases will benefit from refitting with a frequent replacement system as this avoids the long-term build-up of care products. Switching to a one-day disposable lens will obviously avoid all potentially noxious elements in care systems.

'3&9 o'clock' staining

Up to 80% of patients wearing rigid lenses on a daily-wear basis exhibit some degree of '3&9' staining, and approximately 15% of subjects demonstrate clinically significant levels. This very characteristic type of corneal staining only occurs in rigid lens wearers and is due to drying of the medial and lateral regions of the peripheral cornea in association with an unstable tear film. The rigid lens acts as a 'bridge' and prevents the upper lid from massaging the tear film into the cornea during the blink, resulting in a rapid (and often instantaneous) break of the tear film following the blink. Patients usually complain of dry, gritty, irritable eyes and a reduced wearing time. They exhibit conjunctival hyperaemia along the horizontal meridian in conjunction with epithelial punctate staining at the 3–4 and 8–9 o'clock positions (Figure 1.17). In extreme cases the patient may develop a pseudopterygium, vascularized limbal keratitis or

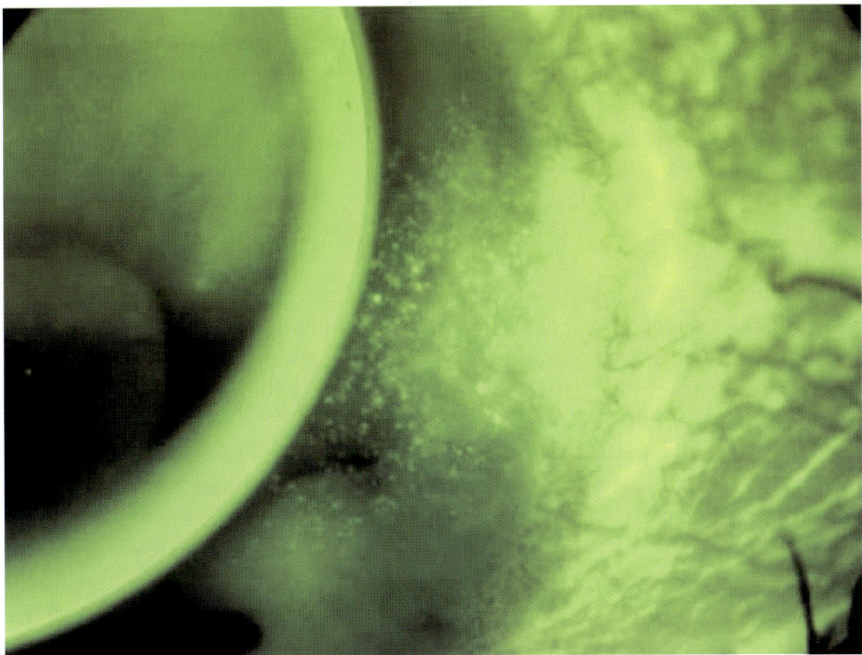

Figure 1.17 Rigid lens-induced '3&9' corneal staining in a patient wearing a high-riding gas-permeable lens with significant peripheral clearance

dellen, in which structural changes to the cornea and adjacent conjunctival tissues occur. The causes are multifactorial and include suboptimal lens fit due to poor centration, small lens size, thick lens edges, excessive edge clearance, inadequate blinking, poor surface wettability and/or abnormal tear composition.

Due to the complex and often multifactorial aetiology of this condition, it is often necessary to deploy numerous simultaneous and/or sequential management strategies to alleviate the problem. Most cases benefit from blinking exercises and artificial lubricants to increase wettability and reduce tear-film drying of the front surface of the lens. Patients with relatively spherical corneas should be fitted with large-diameter lenses with a thin overall thickness profile, thin edge and low edge clearance. Excessively high or low centring lenses should be avoided. This may require the front optic zone diameter to be reduced in high-riding minus lenses and a parallel or negative carrier to be fitted to a low-riding plus lens in order to improve lens centration. If significant corneal astigmatism exists and the lens is decentring as a result of this then a fully back surface toric lens with a large overall diameter and minimal edge clearance should be fitted. In cases where the lens fit and blink rate have been optimized and artificial lubricants instilled – but significant 3&9 o'clock staining persists – the final resort may be to refit the patient with a soft lens. In minor cases of 3&9 o'clock staining the prognosis is excellent. In severe cases total elimination of the staining may be impossible (without resorting to a soft lens) and reduction of the staining to a clinically acceptable level may be the best possible outcome (Businger *et al.*, 1989; Grohe and Lebow, 1989; Campbell and Caroline, 1995; Schnider *et al.*, 1996; Schnider *et al.*, 1997; Davis and Lebow, 2000).

Mechanical staining
Rigid lens wearers may exhibit corneal staining due to a variety of mechanical causes, the most common of which is the presence of a foreign body trapped beneath the lens. Patients exhibit a classical foreign body tracking pattern (Figure 1.18) and the situation is initially managed by removing the lens. The lens is rinsed and the eye thoroughly checked to ensure that the offending object is not trapped under the upper lid. In most instances, except where severe corneal staining has occurred, the lens may be immediately reinserted. Other causes of mechanical staining include lens edge defects (Efron and Veys, 1992), a bound lens and dimple-veil pooling. Bound lenses, typically following overnight wear, occur due to the lens being 'glued' to the cornea by the mucous layer of the tear film. The management of lens binding is somewhat controversial (Swarbrick and Holden, 1996). In most cases, fitting a smaller, more mobile lens on a frequent replace-

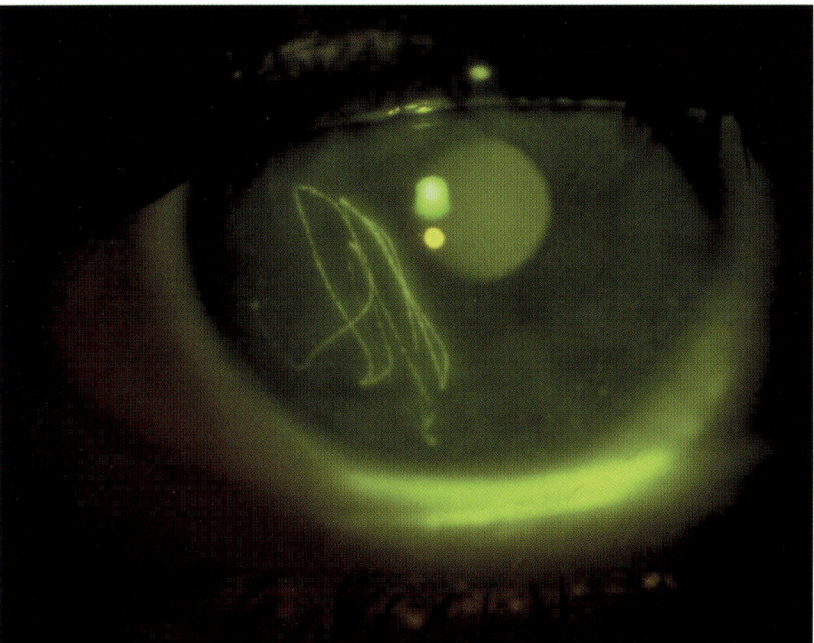

Figure 1.18 Corneal staining from a foreign body trapped under a rigid lens. The abraded areas are clearly observed due to the uptake of fluorescein

ment basis (Woods and Efron, 1996) will alleviate the problem. Dimple-veil 'staining' is not true staining, in that fluorescein is not taken up by the corneal tissue; instead, fluorescein pools in indentations in the epithelial surface. This condition is caused by air bubbles becoming trapped between the back surface of the lens and the corneal epithelium (Figure 1.19) and is due to a poor lens–cornea fitting relationship (Jones and Jones, 1995). It is usually observed centrally in steep-fitting rigid lenses or peripherally in high-riding lenses in cases of high with-the-rule astigmatism. Patients are asymptomatic and the indentations in the corneal epithelium are similar in appearance to the stippled surface of a golf ball. Improving the fitting relationship will immediately eliminate the signs.

Stromal changes

The corneal stroma is not susceptible to direct mechanical insult; however, this corneal layer displays significant changes in thickness when the cornea is made hypoxic, and can suffer a temporary or permanent loss of clarity as a result of various infectious processes.

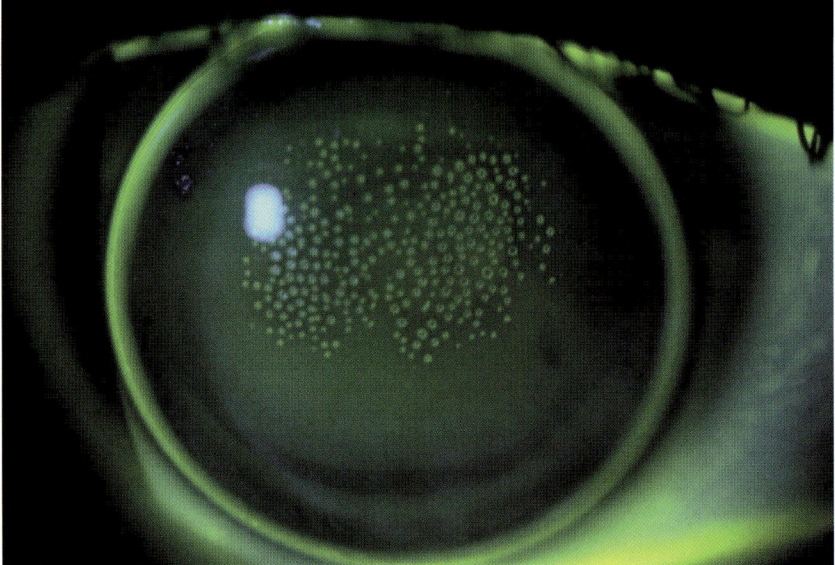

Figure 1.19 Central dimple-veil in a patient wearing a rigid lens which is steep centrally

Hypoxia

The corneal stroma requires only a modest supply of oxygen because the only metabolically active elements of note within this layer are the keratocytes. Although the stroma is dependent upon the atmosphere for this corneal oxygen supply, it displays marked changes when the anterior corneal surface is made hypoxic because of the indirect effects of epithelial hypoxia. Specifically, hypoxia of the epithelium causes this tissue to respire anaerobically, which produces excess lactate. This lactate diffuses into the stroma, creating an osmotic load that leads to corneal swelling. Clear signs of stromal oedema can be detected using the slit lamp.

Striae

The average minimum oxygen transmissibility (Dk/t) to maintain normal corneal metabolism is 24×10^{-9} $(cm/s) \times (ml\,O_2/ml \times mmHg)$ for daily wear and 87×10^{-9} $(cm/s) \times (ml\,O_2/ml \times mmHg)$ for extended wear (Holden and Mertz, 1984; Holden et al., 1984). If contact lenses are unable to provide this level of oxygen then the cornea becomes oxygen-deficient, it begins to respire anaerobically, and becomes hypoxic (Bonnano and Polse, 1992). Hypoxia causes an accumulation of lactic acid in the cornea, resulting in an osmotic shift within the stroma and subsequent fluid entry into the cornea ('oedema'). Once the level of oedema reaches 5% then fine vertically oriented lines are observed in the posterior stroma (Figure 1.20). These are termed 'striae' and are believed to be due to disruption of the regularly packed collagen fibres within the stroma (Polse and Mandell, 1976). The number of striae proportionally increases with increasing oedema (La Hood and Grant, 1990).

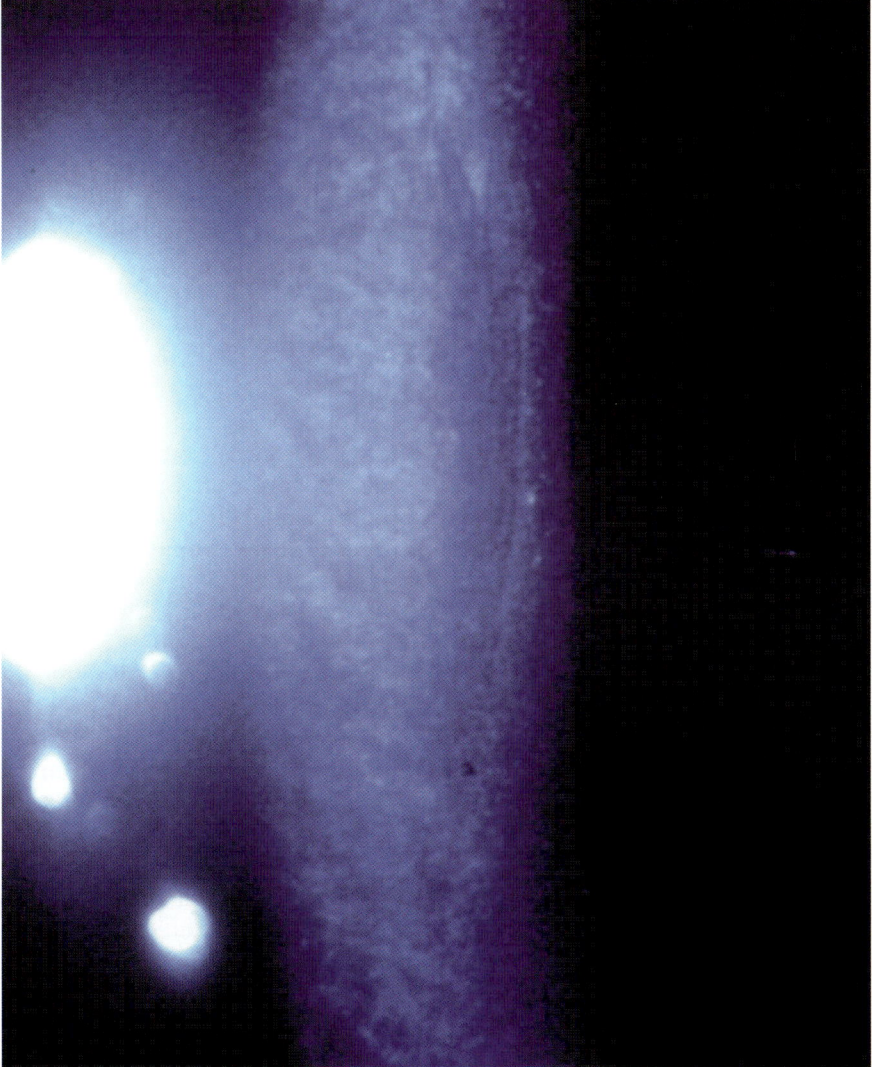

Figure 1.20 Stromal striae due to excessive corneal oedema (Courtesy of Steve Zantos)

Folds

Once the level of oedema reaches 8% then darker lines are observed in the posterior stroma ('folds'). These probably represent a physical buckling of the posterior stromal layers in response to high levels of oedema. This condition is easily managed by increasing the level of oxygen supplied to the cornea, either by reducing lens wear time or increasing the oxygen transmissibility of the lens.

Inflammation

The corneal response that occurs following exposure to an inflammatory stimulus is the development of corneal infiltrates. Corneal infiltrates are focal accumulations of inflammatory cells (polymorphonuclear leuco-cytes, macrophages and lymphocytes) that have entered the cornea from the limbal vasculature as a result of an inflammatory response (Gordon and Kracher, 1985; Silbert, 2000). Infiltrates can be observed in the cornea and/or limbus as regions of intra-epithelial, subepithelial or stromal haze. They may be observed in a wide variety of presentations, ranging from a single focus in an otherwise white eye (with an intact epithelium) to multiple foci in an inflamed, hyperaemic eye, with or without an overlying epithelial defect (Josephson *et al.*, 1988).

The chemotactic stimulus to leucocyte invasion in non-lens wearers includes trauma, and allergic, toxic and viral causes, and any patient presenting with corneal infiltrates should be promptly and carefully assessed to investigate the most likely cause. The appropriate treatment of such a condition depends upon the correct aetiology being ascertained. The stimuli for the development of corneal infiltrates associated with contact lens wear are numerous, and include hypoxia, solution pre-servative toxicity and hypersensitivity, retrolens debris, bacterial con-tamination of lenses and a tightly fitting lens (Hood, 1994; Willcox *et al.*, 1995; Efron, 1997; Donshik, 1998; Swarbrick and Holden, 2000).

The primary concern with any patient presenting with a 'white patch' within the cornea, photophobia and irritation, is to decide if the infiltrate is 'sterile' or 'infected', as the management of such cases will be significantly different. Due to the complexities and time involved in obtaining accurate results from cultures, the differential diagnosis is often undertaken using a clinical signs and symptoms 'model', such as that summarized in Table 1.4 (Stapleton *et al.*, 1993; Grant *et al.*, 1998).

Sterile infiltrates occur in 1% of non-lens wearers and 2–10% of lens wearers. The incidence is higher with soft lens wearers (particularly those using their lenses on an extended-wear basis) and a higher incidence occurs in smokers (Cutter *et al.*, 1996). Among soft lens wearers, microbial keratitis occurs in 0.04% of those wearing lenses on a daily-wear basis and 0.2% of those wearing lenses on an extended-wear basis (Dart, 1993).

Table 1.4 Clinical differentiation between sterile and infective infiltrates

'Presumed' sterile	*'Presumed' infective*
An inflammatory response	An infective process
Peripheral/mid-peripheral lesion	Paracentral/central lesion
Lesions 1–2 mm	Lesions >1.5 mm
Circular appearance	Irregular appearance
Mild pain/foreign body sensation	Increasing pain; may be severe
Epithelium – intact or overlying stain	Epithelial staining overlying the infiltrate
Mild ephiphora	Intense epiphora
Mild to moderate injection	Moderate to severe injection
Anterior stroma involved only	Anterior to mid-stromal involvement
Mild (if any) corneal suppuration	Severe, progressive corneal suppuration
Minimal anterior chamber reaction	Anterior chamber flare and occasional hypopyon

Occasionally, patients are asymptomatic; however, the majority report a minor foreign body sensation, mild discomfort, photophobia and lacrimation (Cutter *et al.*, 1996). On slit lamp examination the conjunctiva is hyperaemic and there is usually an area of bulbar limbal dilation which clearly 'points' to the area of infiltrates (Figure 1.21). The cornea exhibits subepithelial focal spots of haziness, normally in the limbal area. These spots may be focal, band-like or diffuse in nature, and can range in appearance from small, hazy grey-white foci to a 'snowball' type appearance. The management will vary depending upon the cause. In most instances the condition is self-limiting if the noxious stimulus is removed, which generally amounts to a temporary cessation of lens wear, and subsequently effecting a change to the lens wear and care regime. In the interim, the simple palliative measure of artificial tears will suffice, with the infiltrates clearing over a 3–5 day period. In severe cases a topical combination drug containing an antibiotic and steroid can prove useful to clear the condition more rapidly. Long-term lid cleansing measures can be introduced as a useful prophylactic measure.

Although there are many causes of infiltrates, the majority of cases observed in contact lens wearers can be divided into the four principal types described below.

Infiltrative keratitis (IK)
Infiltrative keratitis is an inflammatory reaction of the cornea that manifests as moderate bulbar redness and stromal infiltration. It can occur with or without epithelial involvement and in some cases the

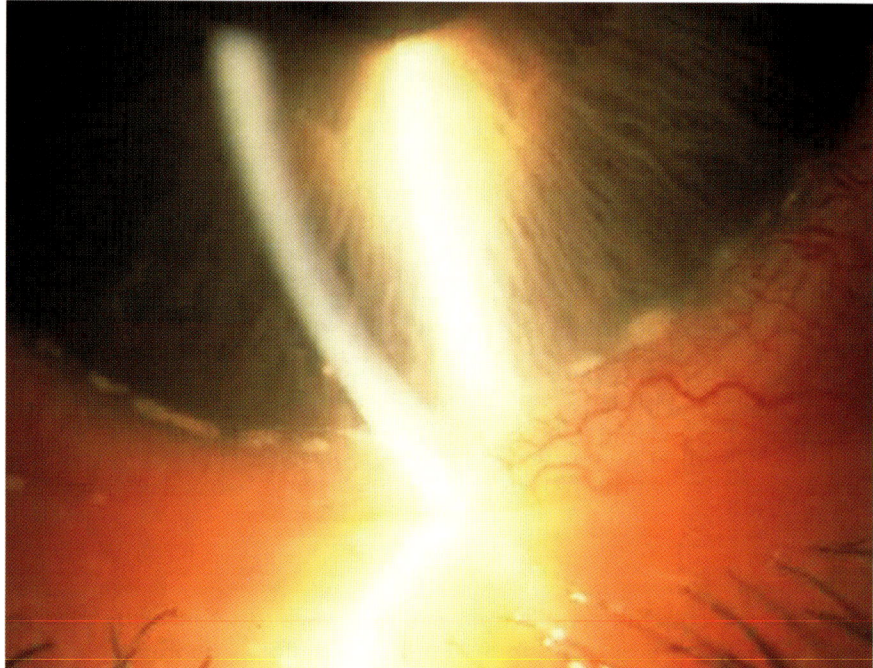

Figure 1.21 Marginal infiltrates in an extended-wear patient (Courtesy of Ian Cox)

cornea may stain with fluorescein. The cornea shows mild to moderate diffuse infiltrates and/or small focal infiltrates that are usually peripherally located in the limbal area. There are many causes (e.g. foreign body trapped beneath a contact lens, mechanical trauma, bacterial toxins, etc.). Infiltrative keratitis occurs in both lens wearers and non-lens wearers, and recent work has shown that the majority of cases are due to Gram-positive exotoxins (in particular *Staphylococcus* spp. and *Streptococcus* spp.) found on the lid margin. This explains the higher incidence of infiltrative keratitis in the 4 and 8 o'clock positions, where the lid lies in apposition with the corneal limbus. The presumed higher incidence in soft lens wearers is due to the toxins being concentrated against the cornea by the hydrogel lens.

Patients are occasionally unaware of any complications – asymptomatic infiltrative keratitis ('AIK') – and the infiltrates are merely noted as an incidental finding during an aftercare examination. The cause of AIK is unknown, but it may be indicative of a low-grade inflammation in response to lens wear or care regimen use. Infiltrative keratitis (IK) occurs in non-lens wearers and in patients wearing both daily-wear and extended-wear lenses. The cornea exhibits focal, non-staining infiltrates;

these may occur anywhere in the cornea, but typically present in the limbal area. Patients with IK report a slight foreign body discomfort and a mild hyperaemia.

Recurrent IK is often related to lid margin disease. Blepharitis is a chronic inflammation of the lid margin that is frequently associated with secondary changes in the conjunctiva and cornea (Smith and Flowers, 1995). While the exact aetiology of blepharitis remains unclear, the presence of *Staphylococcus aureus* and *Staph. epidermidis* is implicated. The presence of staphylococci may result in blepharitis due to direct infection of the lids, a reaction to staphylococcal exotoxin, or an allergic reaction to staphylococcal antigens. Recurrent and long-term chronic inflammatory changes result in notching and thickening of the lid margin (tylosis), loss of lashes (madarosis), white lashes (poliosis) and misdirected lashes (trichiasis). Untreated anterior blepharitis can ultimately result in several corneal complications. A punctate epithelial keratopathy frequently develops in the inferior third of the cornea, possibly as a result of a toxic reaction to staphylococcal exotoxins or destabilization of the tear film. Patients with long-standing blepharitis frequently develop peripheral corneal infiltrates in the 4 and 8 o'clock positions as a hypersensitivity reaction to staphylococcal antigens. In such conditions, lid scrubs and hot compresses are the mainstay of treatment (Fisch, 1991), possibly in combination with the application of an antibiotic ointment with efficacy against staphylococci, such as bacitracin and erythromycin (Everett *et al.*, 1993). Blepharitis is a chronic condition that will recur if left untreated.

Management of IK in a contact lens wearer commences with discontinuation of lens wear until full resolution of all corneal staining occurs. The patient should be monitored carefully over the first 24 hours, but in many cases no medication is required. Severe cases may benefit from a topical antibiotic, primarily to prevent secondary infection due to the fact that the corneal barrier function has been compromised. All cases require attention to lid hygiene, and patients should be immediately placed on an intensive course of warm compresses and lid scrubs. In the long term, there may be a small residual scar, depending upon the aetiology and depth of penetration of the infiltrate.

Contact lens peripheral ulcer (CLPU)

CLPU is often considered to be synonymous with culture negative peripheral ulcer (CNPU); this is not strictly true, as any sterile infiltrate is by definition a CNPU, whereas CLPU is a distinct clinical entity related specifically to contact lens wear (typically extended wear). Contact lens peripheral ulcer is due to corneal exposure to high numbers of pathogenic Gram-positive bacteria (Willcox *et al.*, 1995). The inflammation is caused by a reaction to staphylococcal toxins and results in a focal, circumscribed, round infiltrate.

The patient complains of mild pain (typically foreign body in nature), mild lacrimation and mild photophobia. The cornea usually exhibits a single peripheral/mid-peripheral lesion that is 0.1–1.5 mm in diameter, circular in appearance (Figure 1.22) and is often positioned beneath the upper lid. The infiltrates stain due to a full-thickness loss of epithelium.

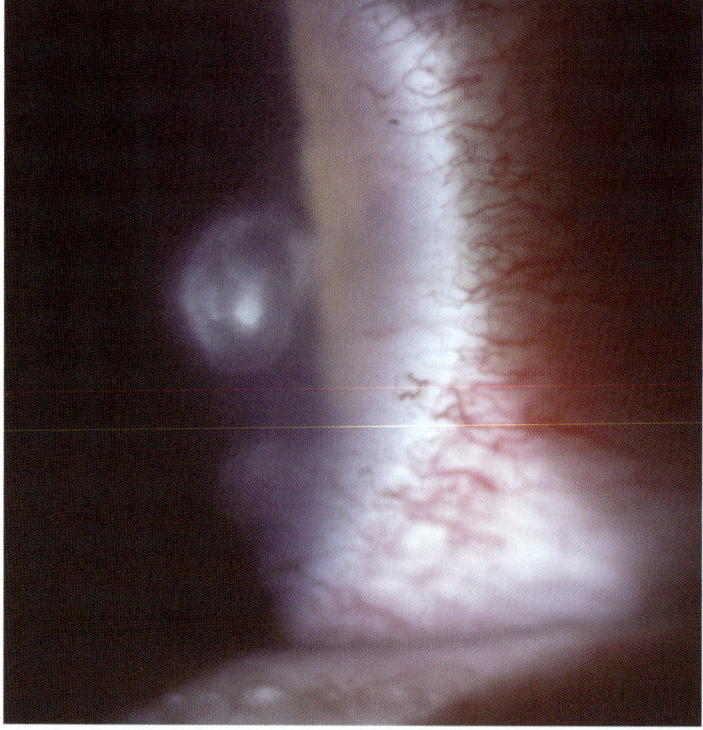

Figure 1.22 CLPU in an extended-wear patient (Courtesy of Michael Hare)

The anterior limiting lamina (Bowman's layer) is intact and the area demonstrates dense infiltration with polymorphonuclear leucocytes (Holden *et al.*, 1999). The condition is self-limiting on removal of the contact lens. Patients should be monitored over the first 24 hours and cease lens wear for 3–14 days. Artificial tears are often beneficial, both to act as a lubricant to prevent the lid rubbing over the epithelial break and also to dilute the bacterial toxin/antigen. Severe cases require a prophylactic antibiotic or combination antibiotic/steroid drug. The condition typically resolves with a single isolated spherical scar. Lid hygiene measures are useful, and there appears to be a patient predisposition, with certain individuals suffering from repeat episodes of the condition. This would be expected in light of the bacterial aetiology, and so those who suffer from repeat episodes should be removed from extended-wear and possibly refitted with rigid lenses, where the potential to concentrate exotoxins is much reduced.

Contact lens-induced acute red eye (CLARE)

This acute inflammatory response occurs exclusively in soft lens extended-wear. It is due to the presence of Gram-negative organisms (e.g. *Pseudomonas* spp.) colonizing the lens or lens case (Holden *et al.*, 1996), possibly in conjunction with a tight lens. The major cause of microbial keratitis is the presence of *Pseudomonas* spp. However, CLARE differs from microbial corneal ulceration as the bacteria implicated adhere only to the contact lens and not to the cornea, as occurs in microbial keratitis. This adherence results in the subsequent recruitment of inflammatory cells. A higher incidence of CLARE occurs during periods when patients have an upper respiratory infection, possibly due to the presence of *Haemophilus influenzae* (Sankaridurg *et al.*, 1996).

Patients are typically woken in the early morning by a moderately painful eye, epiphora and photophobia. The corneal infiltrates rarely stain, rapidly resolve and are usually positioned in all quadrants, close to the limbus. There is an associated marked conjunctival hyperaemia (Figure 1.23) and a high number of patients suffer a recurrence of the condition.

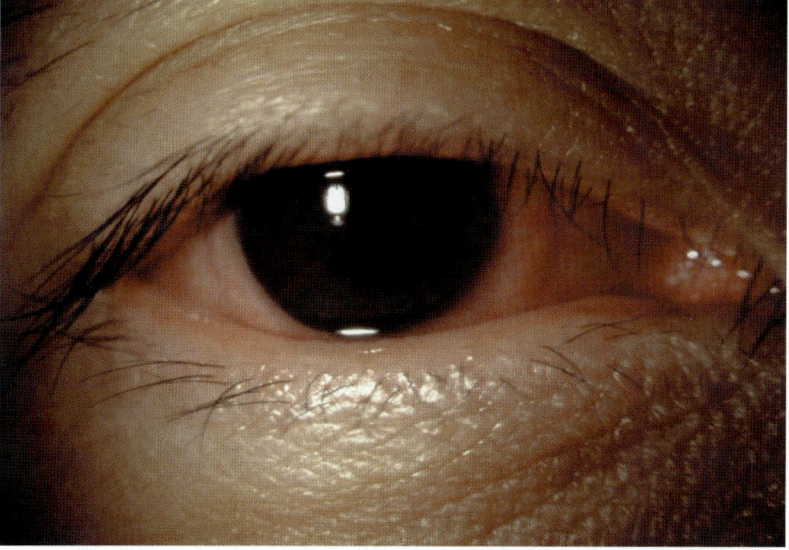

Figure 1.23 CLARE reaction in an extended-wear soft lens-wearing subject. The lens is still *in situ* and the intense conjunctival hyperaemia is clearly seen

Management includes lid hygiene measures, attention to hygiene compliance, refitting with a looser lens and/or a change to daily wear. Due to the influence of *Haemophilus* spp., patients using extended-wear lenses should be advised to switch to daily wear when they have a cold or generally feel unwell.

Adenoviral keratitis

Epidemic keratoconjunctivitis (EKC) occurs due to exposure to human adenovirus, principally serotypes 7, 8, 10, 19, 29 and 37. It usually occurs in adults and is bilateral in 60% of cases. There is typically a history of an upper respiratory tract infection, but no systemic problems. Some 80% of sufferers develop a diffuse, central subepithelial keratitis, with an acute onset of a watery discharge, discomfort and photophobia. Tarsal follicles are present and there is usually a tender, palpable pre-auricular lymph node. The condition progresses for 4–7 days and spontaneous resolution of the conjunctivitis occurs in approximately 2 weeks. Treatment in this case consists of palliative measures (artificial tears and cold compresses) and advice to the patient concerning the highly contagious nature of the disease during the initial 2 weeks (Buehler *et al.*, 1984; Murrah, 1988). Patients should be instructed to avoid touching their eyes, to wash their hands frequently, to use disposable towels, and to avoid group activities for as long as an ocular discharge is present (Weber and Eichenbaum, 1997). The use of topical steroids to reduce the inflammatory process is controversial (Pineda and Dohlman, 1994) and is indicated only if the corneal infiltrates significantly reduce vision and a pseudomembrane is present. Recent publications (e.g. Gordon *et al.*, 1998) suggest that topical non-steroidal anti-inflammatory drugs (NSAIDs) may be as good as topical steroids in helping to rehabilitate patients with EKC, but without the potential side-effects. The subepithelial infiltrates usually resolve over a period of months, but may persist for years, in some cases being severe enough to require lamellar keratoplasty (Hanna *et al.*, 1991).

Endothelial changes

Changes in the endothelium induced by contact lens wear are due to the combined effects of hypoxia and hypercapnia. Contact lenses have a minimal mechanical influence on the cornea. The two primary contact lens-induced changes are polymegethism and bleb formations.

Polymegethism

Polymegethism is a term used to describe an endothelial condition in which the ratio of the smallest to largest endothelial cells increases from approximately 1:5 to 1:20 and the endothelium is seen to include cells of significantly differing sizes, when viewed using specular reflection (Figure 1.24), (Doughty and Fonn, 1993). Endothelial changes are a natural process of ageing, but contact lenses accelerate the process and the degree of polymegethism is related to the duration of lens wear and the degree of hypoxia and hypercapnia present (Bergmanson and Weissman, 1992). Specifically, contact lens-induced polymegethism is believed to be due to chronic stromal acidosis caused by long-term hypoxia and hypercapnia, producing a structural reorientation of the endothelial cells (Schoessler and Woloshak, 1981; Holden *et al.*, 1985). This condition may result in a loss of endothelial pump function. Although patients are usually asymptomatic, polymegethism may be linked to the development of a chronic intolerance to lens wear ('corneal exhaustion syndrome') (Sweeney, 1992). Progression of the condition can be arrested by refitting the patient with high gas transmissibility lenses. Prognosis for full recovery is poor, as the endothelial appearance never fully recovers (Holden *et al.*, 1985; McMahon *et al.*, 1996).

Blebs

Approximately 10 minutes after inserting a contact lens, almost 100% of neophyte contact lens wearers exhibit black, non-reflecting areas within the endothelial mosaic that simulate 'holes' in the endothelium (Zantos and Holden, 1977). These 'holes' (or 'blebs') peak after 20–30 minutes and then subside after 2–3 hours. The level of the response is proportional to the lens transmissibility and reduces in adapted wearers, suggesting an adaptive response. This response is believed to be due to endothelial cell oedema caused by a local acidic pH shift (stromal acidosis) as a result of either an increase in carbonic acid through retardation of carbon dioxide efflux (hypercapnia) and/or an increase of lactic acid due to oxygen deprivation (hypoxia) (Bonnano and Polse, 1987). Bulging of the endothelial cells in the direction of the aqueous produces an optically empty area when the cells are viewed in specular reflection. Patients are asymptomatic and no management is required, as the blebs disappear within minutes of lens removal (Efron, 1996b).

Limbal changes

Although the limbus may be considered to be a tissue that is anatomically distinct from the cornea, it is pertinent to consider contact lens-induced limbal changes because these can directly affect the neighbouring cornea, which is the subject of this book. The key morphological distinction

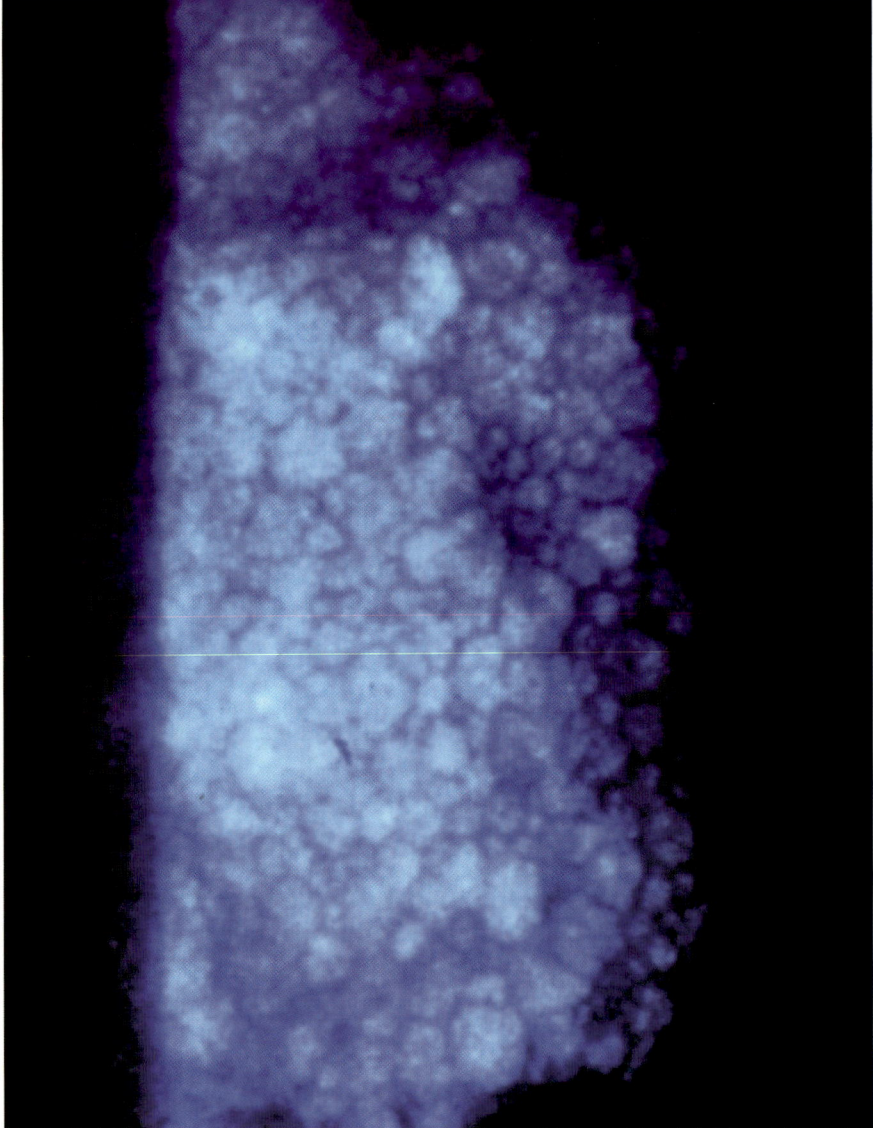

Figure 1.24 Endothelial polymegethism (Courtesy of Steve Zantos)

between the cornea and limbus is that the limbus is the region of the corneal stem cells, transitional tissue and blood vessels. As a result of the last of these features in particular, the limbus is capable of supporting a wide range of pathological events – far more than the cornea is capable of – that are mediated by blood vessels.

Hypoxia

In all tissues of the body, hypoxia serves as a stimulus to vascular engorgement and proliferation. While such mechanisms can be potentially beneficial elsewhere in the body (e.g. to bring more oxygen to hypoxic tissues), they are detrimental to the cornea because of the potential for blood vessels to cover the pupil and interfere with vision. Perhaps of less immediate significance from an ocular pathology standpoint – but nevertheless important to contact lens wearers – is the unsightly 'red eye' that results from excess limbal hyperaemia.

Limbal hyperaemia

Limbal hyperaemia is very common in wearers of all contact lens types, particularly soft lenses (Figure 1.25). The fact that virtually all lens wearers exhibit some degree of limbal hyperaemia highlights the necessity of recording accurate baseline values of this sign. Patients are invariably asymptomatic and exhibit engorgement of the limbal blood vessels. Recent work has suggested that limbal hyperaemia is predominantly due to the

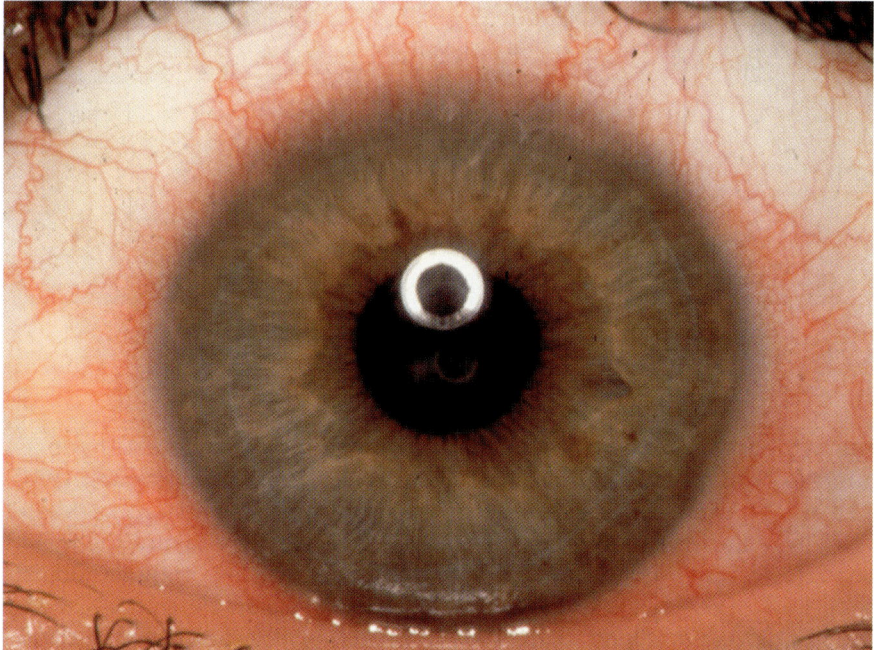

Figure 1.25 Severe limbal hyperaemia produced through the long-term use of low-permeability soft lenses on an extended-wear schedule (Courtesy of Desmond Fonn)

presence of subclinical levels of hypoxia (Papas *et al.*, 1997; Papas, 1998). In minor cases no treatment is necessary, but chronic cases may be linked to subsequent neovascular changes within the cornea (McMonnies, 1984). Management options include reducing lens wearing time, substantially increasing lens transmissibility and/or optimizing the lens fit.

Corneal vascularization

The 'normal' cornea is avascular and the development of corneal vascularization (Figure 1.26) is a complex event. Potential causes of new vessel growth in a previously avascular cornea (vascularization) linked to

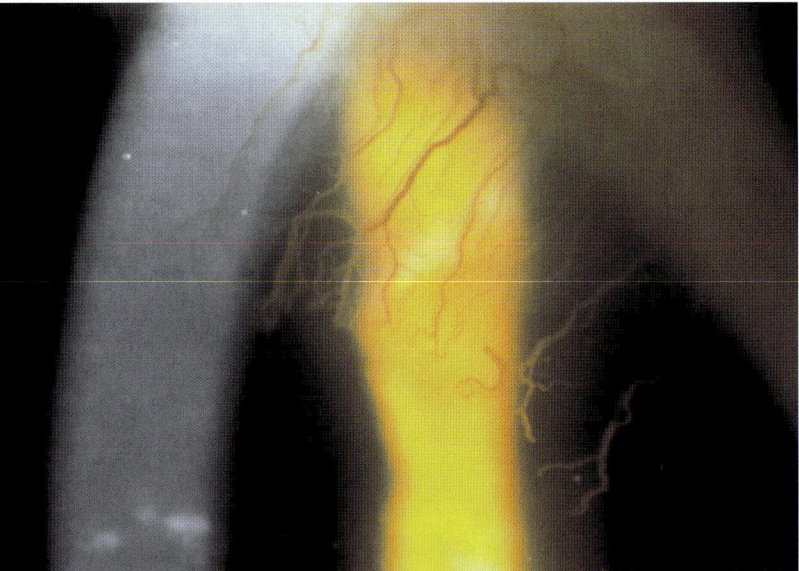

Figure 1.26 Substantial corneal vascularization in a soft-lens wearer (Courtesy of Patrick Caroline)

contact lens wear include solution hypersensitivity, trauma and hypoxia, and the process may be linked to limbal hyperaemia (McMonnies, 1984). The major problem associated with determining the extent of vessel growth relates to the reference point from which to measure the vessel change. The degree of vascularization is related to lens transmissibility, with <1% of rigid lens wearers, 5–10% of daily-wear soft and 10–20% of extended-wear soft lens wearers exhibiting clinically significant vascularization (Efron, 1996a). The degree of vessel ingrowth is usually greater in the superior cornea, as a result of the reduction in oxygenation beneath the upper lid. The true aetiology of vascularization is complex, but it would appear that hypoxia produces stromal oedema and softening, and the subsequent release of vasostimulatory agents results in the ingrowth of vessels into the cornea (Efron, 1987). Although patients are asymptomatic, corneal vascularization must be avoided as vessel ingrowth can lead to subsequent visual loss due to inflammation and lipid deposition. Also, a patient may not be able to opt for refractive surgery at some later stage if the limbal vascular ingrowth is too extensive. The management in severe cases of vascularization is to significantly increase corneal oxygenation by increasing lens transmissibility and/or reducing wearing time. The prognosis for recovery from vascularization is excellent, although residual 'ghost' vessels in the cornea may remain many months or even years after refitting.

Staining

The limbus is susceptible to two pathological changes that both occur superiorly – superior limbic keratoconjunctivitis (SLK) and superior epithelial arcuate lesions (SEALS). Although the latter condition is not strictly a limbal condition, it is best considered here because it does occur in the proximity of the limbus and similar techniques are required to observe both conditions.

Superior limbic keratoconjunctivitis (SLK)

SLK may be idiopathic or occur secondary to soft contact lens wear (CL-SLK) (Stenson, 1983). In the idiopathic form, SLK is often seen in middle-aged females with thyroid dysfunction (Theodore, 1963). Symptoms of CL-SLK include contact lens intolerance, burning, itching and photophobia (Stenson, 1983). Initially the superior cornea shows a superficial punctate keratitis. If left untreated the superior bulbar conjunctiva demonstrates fluorescein staining and the superior lid develops papillary hypertrophy. Further changes include bilateral epithelial dulling, formation of subepithelial opacities and infiltrates, and marked punctate staining of the upper one- to two-thirds of the cornea. Finally a V-shaped fibrovascular pannus forms at the superior limbus; the pannus consists of vascularized connective tissue. If left unchecked, this condition may progress to result in visual loss. Contact lens-induced superior limbic keratoconjunctivitis is frequently associated with daily wear hydrogel lenses disinfected with thimerosal solutions (Binder et al., 1981). Other suggested causes include atopic/allergic complications (Stenson, 1983) and mechanical irritation (Abel et al., 1985).

Treatment of CL-SLK consists of discontinuation of contact lenses and eventual refitting with RGP lenses or frequent replacement/disposable soft lenses without exposure to thimerosal-preserved disinfectants. The presence of SLK requires referral to a medical practitioner for evaluation of the thyroid function of the patient.

Superior epithelial arcuate lesions staining

Splits in the superior epithelium secondary to contact lens wear are commonly termed SEALS (Hine *et al.*, 1987). An area of deep staining is seen approximately 1 mm from the superior limbus between 10 o'clock and 2 o'clock (Figure 1.27). The staining is arcuate in shape, runs parallel

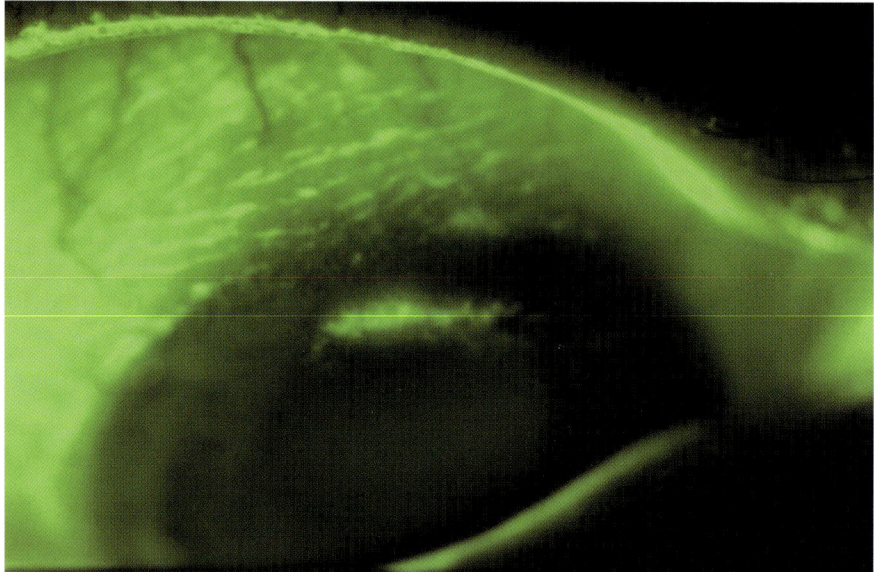

Figure 1.27 Superior epithelial arcuate lesion obtained following the use of a thick, high water content lens

to the limbus, and is 0.1–0.3 mm wide and 2–5 mm in length. This condition is normally unilateral and usually asymptomatic, although patients occasionally complain of a slight foreign body sensation under the lid that is often worse upon lens removal. This may be because the lens acts as a 'bandage', preventing the upper lid from abrading the split area of the epithelium. The problem occasionally resolves spontaneously once a period of non-lens wear occurs, although it often requires a change in lens material or design.

The causative mechanism behind the problem is poorly understood, with mechanical factors, solutions effects, hypoxia and dehydration all being implicated in some way (Hine *et al.*, 1987; Malinovsky *et al.*, 1989;

Young and Mirejovsky, 1993; Holden *et al.*, 2001). Of these possibilities, the most compelling argument is that SEALS is caused by mechanical trauma induced by the inflexible nature of some hydrogel lenses (Young and Mirejovsky, 1993) and silicone hydrogel lenses (Holden *et al.*, 2001).

Soft lenses align the central cornea by steepening from their nominal base-curve and then rapidly flattening beyond the limbus to align the sclera. This requires the hydrogel material to adopt an 'S' shape. If a material is too thick or has a high elastic modulus then the material will be forced into a compromise 'S' shape that will not perfectly align the limbal area. The greatest misalignment will occur in the superior corneal periphery due to the pressure induced by the upper lid, which results in mechanical irritation. Under normal conditions the post-lens tear film acts as a lubricant to prevent the lens 'rubbing' against the corneal epithelium. However, in such cases as these the eyelid forces the tears out from between the misaligned lens and the corneal area immediately adjacent to it, resulting in frictional forces between the lens and cornea and subsequent arcuate epithelial insult. The increased rigidity and relative inflexibility of the new silicone-hydrogel lens materials compared with conventional hydrogel materials explains why such materials may be more prone to induce SEAL staining than conventional materials (Holden *et al.*, 2000).

To alleviate the problem, patients should cease lens wear for 3–4 days. In approximately one-third of patients, the problem will spontaneously resolve and not recur (Hine *et al.*, 1987). If the problem does recur then a change in lens type/design is required to increase the flexibility of the material and/or increase the peripheral lens alignment. In most cases, refitting with a thinner, more flexible lens material and/or changing to a lens of flatter radius of the same design, will alleviate the problem. Switching to mid-water content disposable or ultra-thin polyHEMA lenses frequently resolves the condition.

Conclusion

Although virtually all of the corneal complications of contact lens wear discussed in this chapter are non-sight-threatening and generally self-limiting, some may progress to cause severe short-term discomfort and visual loss and may compromise the integrity of the cornea and render it susceptible to more serious problems. An example is contact lens-induced hypoxic corneal staining, which if left unchecked increases the risk of developing a chance infectious keratitis. Clearly, early identification of such problems and appropriate action by the practitioner will make contact lens wear more safe, enjoyable and comfortable for our patients.

This chapter has outlined the application of the slit lamp for the examination of contact lens-related corneal disorders, as well as providing an overview of the clinical manifestations of these conditions. The information presented in Chapter 2 by Weissman and Mondino will complement this information, and Chapters 3 and 4 will outline how *in vivo* confocal microscopy and *in vitro* light and electron microscopy has expanded and strengthened our understanding of contact lens-related corneal disorders beyond the conventional clinical setting.

Acknowledgements

The authors would like to acknowledge Jane Veys, Philippe Betran and Ian Davies for their invaluable assistance in compiling this chapter, in addition to those who very kindly allowed their pictures to be reproduced.

References

Abel, R., Shovlin, J. P. and DePaolis, M. D. (1985) A treatise on hydrophilic lens induced superior limbic keratoconjunctivitis. *Int. Contact Lens Clin.*, **12**, 116–123.

Abelson, M. B. and Holly, F. J. (1977) A tentative mechanism for inferior punctate keratopathy. *Am. J. Ophthalmol.*, **83**, 866–869.

Atkins, N. and Allsopp, G. (1996). Multi-purpose solution intolerance – diagnosis and management. *Optician*, **212**(5562), 22–31.

Back, A. (1988) Corneal staining with contact lens wear. *J. Br. Contact Lens Assoc. Trans. Ann. Clin. Conf.*, 16–18.

Bailey, I. L., Bullimore, M. A., Raasch, T. W. *et al.* (1991) Clinical grading and the effects of scaling. *Invest. Ophthalmol. Vis. Sci.*, **32**, 422–432.

Begley, C. G., Barr, J. T., Edrington, T. B. *et al.* (1996) Characteristics of corneal staining in hydrogel contact lens wearers. *Optom. Vis. Sci.*, **73**, 193–200.

Bergmanson, J. P. G. and Weissman, B. A. (1992) Hypoxic changes in corneal endothelium. In *Complications of Contact Lens Wear.* (A. Tomlinson, ed.), pp. 37–67, Mosby Year Book.

Binder, P. S., Rasmussen, D. M. and Gordon, M. (1981) Keratoconjunctivitis and soft lens solutions. *Arch. Ophthalmol.*, **99**, 87–90.

Bonnano, J. and Polse, K. (1992) Hypoxic changes in the corneal epithelium and stroma. In *Complications of Contact Lens Wear.* (A. Tomlinson, ed.), pp. 21–36, Mosby Year Book.

Bonnano, J. A. and Polse, K. A. (1987) Corneal acidosis during contact lens wear: effects of hypoxia and CO_2. *Invest. Ophthalmol. Vis. Sci.*, **28**, 1514–1520.

Bowen, K. P. (1993) Slit lamp photography. *Spectrum*, **8**(7), 27–33.

Brennan, N. A., Efron, N., Bruce, A. S. *et al.* (1988) Dehydration of hydrogel lenses: Environmental influences during normal wear. *Am. J. Optom. Physiol. Opt.*, **65**, 277–281.

Buehler, J. W., Finton, R. J., Goodman, R. A. *et al.* (1984) Epidemic keratoconjunctivitis: report of an outbreak in an ophthalmology practice and recommendations for prevention. *Infect. Control*, **5**, 390–394.

Businger, U., Treiber, A. and Flury, C. (1989) The aetiology and management of three and nine o'clock staining. *Int. Contact Lens Clin.*, **16**, 136–139.

Caffery, B. E. and Josephson, J. E. (2000) Complications of lens care solution. In *Anterior Segment Complications of Contact Lens Wear*, 2nd edn (J. A. Silbert, ed.), pp. 149–163, Butterworth-Heinemann.

Campbell, R. and Caroline, P. (1995) Dellen formation in RGP contact lens patients. *Spectrum*, **10**(6), 56.

CCLRU (1997) CCLRU grading scales (Appendix D). In *Contact Lenses*, 4th edn (A. J. Phillips and L. Speedwell, eds), pp. 863–867, Butterworth-Heinemann.

Collins, M. J., Stahmer, D. and Pearson, G. (1989) Clinical findings associated with incomplete blinking in soft lens wearers. *Clin. Exp. Optom.*, **72**, 55–60.

Courtney, R. C. and Lee, J. M. (1982) Predicting ocular intolerance of a contact lens solution by use of a filter system enhancing fluorescein staining detection. *Int. Contact Lens Clin.*, **9**(5), 302–310.

Cox, I. (1995) Digital imaging in the contact lens practice. *Int. Contact Lens Clin.*, **22**(3/4), 62–66.

Cox, I. and Fonn, D. (1991) Interference filters to eliminate the surface reflex and improve contrast during fluorescein photography. *Int. Contact Lens Clin.*, **18**(9/10), 178–181.

Cutter, G. R., Chalmers, R. L. and Roseman, M. (1996) The clinical presentation, prevalence and risk factors of focal corneal infiltrates in soft contact lens wearers. *Contact Lens Assoc. Ophthalmol. J.*, **22**, 30–37.

Dart, J. K. G. (1993) The epidemiology of contact lens related disease in the United Kingdom. *Contact Lens Assoc. Ophthalmol. J.*, **19**, 241–246.

Davis, L. J. and Lebow, K. A. (2000) Noninfectious corneal staining. In *Anterior Segment Complications of Contact Lens Wear*, 2nd edn (J. A. Silbert, ed.), pp. 67–93, Butterworth-Heinemann.

Donshik, P. (1998) Peripheral corneal infiltrates and contact lens wear. *Contact Lens Assoc. Ophthalmol. J.*, **24**, 134–136.

Dougal, J. (1992) Abrasions secondary to contact lens wear. In *Complications of Contact Lens Wear* (A. Tomlinson, ed.), pp. 123–156, Mosby Year Book.

Doughty, M. J. and Fonn, D. (1993) Pleomorphism and endothelial cell size in normal and polymegethous human corneal endothelium. *Int. Contact Lens Clin.*, **20**(5/6), 116–122.

Efron, N. (1987) Vascular response of the cornea to contact lens wear. *J. Am. Optom. Assoc.*, **58**, 836–846.

Efron, N. (1996a) Contact lens induced corneal neovascularisation. *Optician*, **211**(5533), 26–35.

Efron, N. (1996b) Contact lens induced endothelial blebs. *Optician*, **212**(5567), 34–37.

Efron, N. (1997) Contact lens-induced sterile infiltrative keratitis. *Optician*, **214**(5608), 16–22.

Efron, N. (1999) *Contact Lens Complications*. Butterworth-Heinemann/Optician.

Efron, N. (2000) *Efron Grading Scales for Contact Lens Complications*, Millennium edn, Butterworth-Heinemann/Optician (available from Hydron UK).

Efron, N. and Veys, J. (1992) Defects in disposable contact lenses can compromise ocular integrity. *Int. Contact Lens Clin.*, **19**, 8–18.

Efron, N., Brennan, N., Bruce, A. *et al.* (1987) Dehydration of hydrogel lenses under normal wearing conditions. *Contact Lens Assoc. Ophthalmol. J.*, **13**, 152–156.

Efron, N., Golding, T. R. and Brennan, N. A. (1991) The effect of soft lens lubricants on symptoms and lens dehydration. *Contact Lens Assoc. Ophthalmol. J.*, **17**, 114–119.

Efron, N., Morgan, P. B. and Katsara, S. S. (2001) Validation of grading scales for contact lens complications. *Ophthal. Physiol. Opt.*, **21**, 17–29.

Everett, S. L., Karenchak, L. M., Kowalski, R. P. *et al.* (1993) Which are the best first-line antibiotics for treating conjunctivitis and blepharitis? *Invest. Ophthalmol. Vis. Sci.*, **34**, S851.

Fisch, B. M. (1991) Clinical management of eyelid disease. *Spectrum*, **6**(2), 40–50.

Gordon, A. and Kracher, G. P. (1985) Corneal infiltrates and extended-wear contact lenses. *J. Am. Optom. Assoc.*, **56**, 198–201.

Gordon, Y. J., Araullo-Cruz, T. and Romanowski, E. G. (1998) The effects of topical nonsteroidal anti-inflammatory drugs on adenoviral replication. *Arch. Ophthalmol.*, **116**, 900–905.

Grant, T., Chong, M. S., Vajdic, C. *et al.* (1998) Contact lens induced peripheral ulcers during hydrogel contact lens wear. *Contact Lens Assoc. Ophthalmol. J.*, **24**, 145–151.

Grimmer, P. R. (1992) Soft contact lens water content and five common post-fitting complications. Are there relationships? *Clin. Exp. Optom.*, **75**, 182–187.

Grohe, R. M. and Lebow, K. A. (1989) Vascularized limbal keratitis. *Int. Contact Lens Clin.*, **16**(7&8), 197–209.

Guillon, M., Guillon, J. P., Styles, E. *et al.* (1995) Corneal staining characteristics for nonwearers and soft contact lens wearers. *Optom. Vis. Sci.*, **72**, S93.

Hammack, G. G. (1995) Updated video equipment recommendations for slit-lamp videography for 1995. *Int. Contact Lens Clin.*, **22**(3/4), 54–61.

Hanna, K. D., Besson, D. T. and Pouliquen, Y. (1991) Lamellar keratoplasty with the Barraquer microkeratome. *J. Refract. Corneal Surg.*, **7**, 177–181.

Helton, D. O. and Watson, L. S. (1991) Hydrogel contact lens dehydration rates determined by thermogravimetric analysis. *Contact Lens Assoc. Ophthalmol. J.*, **17**, 59–61.

Henson, D. B. (1996) Slit lamps. In *Optometric Instrumentation* (D. Henson, ed.), pp. 138–161, Butterworth-Heinemann.

Hine, N., Back, A. and Holden, B. A. (1987) Aetiology of arcuate epithelial lesions induced by hydrogels. *J. Br. Contact Lens Assoc. Trans. Ann. Clin. Conf.*, 48–50.

Holden, B. A. and Mertz, G. W. (1984) Critical oxygen levels to avoid corneal edema for daily and extended wear contact lenses. *Invest. Ophthalmol. Vis. Sci.*, **25**, 1161–1167.

Holden, B. A. and Sweeney, D. F. (1991) The significance of the microcyst response: a review. *Optom. Vis. Sci.*, **68**, 703–707.

Holden, B. A., Sweeney, D. F. and Sanderson, G. (1984) The minimum precorneal oxygen tension to avoid corneal edema. *Invest. Ophthalmol. Vis. Sci.*, **25**, 476–480.

Holden, B. A., Sweeney, D. F., Vannas, A. *et al.* (1985) Effects of long-term extended contact lens wear on the human cornea. *Invest. Ophthalmol. Vis. Sci.*, **26**, 1489–1501.

Holden, B. A., La Hood, D., Grant, T. *et al.* (1996) Gram negative bacteria can induce contact lens related acute red eye (CLARE) responses. *Contact Lens Assoc. Ophthalmol. J.*, **22**, 47–52.

Holden, B. A., Reddy, M. K., Sankaridurg, P. R. *et al.* (1999) Contact lens-induced peripheral ulcers with extended wear of disposable hydrogel lenses: histopathologic observations on the nature and type of corneal infiltrate. *Cornea*, **18**, 538–543.

Holden, B. A., Sankaridurg, P. R. and Jalbert, I. (2000) Adverse events and infections: which ones and how many? In *Silicone Hydrogels: The Rebirth of Continuous Wear Contact Lenses*. (D. F. Sweeney, ed.), pp. 150–213, Butterworth-Heinemann.

Holden, B. A., Stephenson, A., Stretton, S. *et al.* (2001) Superior epithelial arcuate lesions with soft contact lens wear. *Optom. Vis. Sci.*, **78**, 9–12.

Hood, D. (1994) Do soft lens solutions cause corneal infiltrates? *Spectrum*, **9**(2), 20–23.

Jalbert, I., Sweeney, D. F. and Holden, B. A. (1999) The characteristics of corneal staining in successful daily and extended disposable contact lens wearers. *Clin. Exp. Optom.*, **82**, 4–10.

Jones, L. and Jones, D. (1995) Dimple-veil staining. *Optician*, **210**(5509), 32.

Jones, L. and Jones, D. (2000) *Common Contact Lens Complications*. Butterworth-Heinemann.

Josephson, J. E. and Caffery, B. E. (1992) Corneal staining characteristics after sequential instillations of fluorescein. *Optom. Vis. Sci.*, **69**, 570–573.

Josephson, J. E., Zantos, S., Caffery, B. E. *et al.* (1988) Differentiation of corneal complications observed in contact lens wearers. *J. Am. Optom. Assoc.*, **59**, 679–685.

Keay, L., Sweeney, D. F., Jalbert, I. *et al.* (2000) Microcyst response to high Dk/t silicone hydrogel contact lenses. *Vis. Sci.*, **77**, 582–585.

Korb, D. R. and Herman, J. P. (1979) Corneal staining subsequent to sequential fluorescein installations. *J. Am. Optom. Assoc.*, **50**, 361–367.

Krasnow, D. (1997) Set up your slit lamp for video and digital capture. *Rev. Optom.*, January 15, pp. 47–52.

LaHood, D. and Grant, T. (1990) Striae and folds as indicators of corneal oedema. *Optom. Vis. Sci.*, **67**, S196.

Little, S. A. and Bruce, A. S. (1994) Postlens tear film depletion associated with inferior arcuate staining in ultrathin hydrogel lens wear. *Optom. Vis. Sci.*, **71**, S53.

Lloyd, M. (1992) Lies, statistics, and clinical significance. *J. Br. Contact Lens Assoc.*, **15**, 67–70.

Lowe, R. (1991) Clinical slitlamp photography – an update. *Clin. Exp. Optom.*, **74**, 125–129.

MacDonald, K. E., Fonn, D., Richter, D. B. *et al.* (1995) Comparison of the physiological response to extended wear of an experimental high Dk soft lens versus a 38% HEMA lens. *Invest. Ophthalmol. Vis. Sci.*, **36**, S310.

Malinovsky, V., Pole, J. J., Pence, N. A. *et al.* (1989) Epithelial splits of the superior cornea in hydrogel contact lens patients. *Int. Contact Lens Clin.*, **16**(9&10), 252–254.

Mandell, R. B. (1987) Slit lamp classification system. *J. Am. Optom. Assoc.*, **58**, 198–201.

McMahon, T. T., Polse, K. A., McNamara, N. *et al.* (1996) Recovery from induced corneal edema and endothelial morphology after long-term contact lens wear. *Optom. Vis. Sci.*, **73**, 184–188.

McMonnies, C. W. (1984) Risk factors in the etiology of contact lens induced corneal vascularization. *Int. Contact Lens Clin.*, **11**, 286–293.

McNally, J. J., Chalmers, R. and Seger, R. (1986) Corneal epithelial disruption with extremely thin hydrogel lenses. *Clin. Exp. Optom.*, **70**, 106–111.

Meyler, J. and Burnett-Hodd, N. (1998) The use of digital image capture in contact lens practice. *Contact Lens Ant. Eye*, **21**, S3–S11.

Mondino, B. J., Salamon, S. M. and Zaidman, G. W. (1982) Allergic and toxic reactions in soft contact lens wearers. *Surv. Ophthalmol.*, **26**, 337–344.

Murrah, W. F. (1988) Epidemic keratoconjunctivitis. *Ann. Ophthalmol.*, **20**, 36–38.

Orsborn, G. N. and Zantos, S. G. (1988) Corneal desiccation staining with thin high water content contact lenses. *Contact Lens Assoc. Ophthalmol. J.*, **14**, 81–85.

Papas, E. B. (1998) On the relationship between soft contact lens oxygen transmissibility and induced limbal hyperaemia. *Exp. Eye Res.*, **67**, 125–131.

Papas, E. B., Vajdic, C., Austen, R. *et al.* (1997) High oxygen-transmissibility soft contact lenses do not induce limbal hyperaemia. *Curr. Eye Res.*, **16**, 942–948.

Phelps-Brown, N. (1991) Ocular photography. *Optician*, **202**(5322), 16–26.

Pineda, R. and Dohlman, C. H. (1994) The role of steroids in the management of *Acanthamoeba* keratitis, fungal keratitis and epidemic keratoconjunctivitis. *Int. Ophthalmol. Clin.*, **34**(3), 19–31.

Polse, K. A. and Mandell, R. B. (1976) Etiology of corneal striae accompanying hydrogel lens wear. *Invest. Ophthalmol. Vis. Sci.*, **15**, 553–556.

Sankaridurg, P. R., Willcox, M. D., Sharma, S. *et al.* (1996) *Haemophilus influenzae* adherent to contact lenses associated with production of acute ocular inflammation. *J. Clin. Microbiol.*, **34**, 2426–2431.

Schnider, C. M., Terry, R. L. and Holden, B. A. (1996) Effect of patient and lens performance characteristics on peripheral corneal desiccation. *J. Am. Optom. Assoc.*, **67**, 144–150.

Schnider, C. M., Terry, R. L. and Holden, B. A. (1997) Effect of lens design on peripheral corneal desiccation. *J. Am. Optom. Assoc.*, **68**, 163–170.

Schoessler, J. and Woloshak, M. (1981) Corneal endothelium in veteran PMMA contact lens wearers. *Int. Contact Lens Clin.*, **8**, 19–25.

Schwallie, J. D., McKenney, C. D., Long, W. D. *et al.* (1997) Corneal staining patterns in normal non-contact lens wearers. *Optom. Vis. Sci.*, **74**, 92–98.

Silbert, J. A. (2000) *Anterior Segment Complications of Contact Lens Wear*, 2nd edn. Butterworth-Heinemann.

Smith, R. E. and Flowers, C. W. (1995) Chronic blepharitis: a review. *Contact Lens Assoc. Ophthalmol. J.*, **21**, 200–207.

Stapleton, F., Dart, J. K. G. and Minassian, D. (1993) Risk factors with contact lens related suppurative keratitis *Contact Lens Assoc. Ophthalmol. J.*, **19**, 204–210.

Stenson, S. (1983) Superior limbic keratoconjunctivitis associated with soft contact lens wear. *Arch. Ophthalmol.*, **101**, 402–404.

Swarbrick, H. A. and Holden, B. A. (1996) Effects of lens parameter variation on rigid gas permeable lens adherence. *Optom. Vis. Sci.*, **73**, 144–155.

Swarbrick, H. and Holden, B. (2000) Complications of Hydrogel Extended Wear Lenses. In *Anterior Segment Complications of Contact Lens Wear*, 2nd edn (J. A. Silbert, ed.), pp. 273–308, Butterworth-Heinemann.

Sweeney, D. F. (1992) Corneal exhaustion syndrome with long-term wear of contact lenses. *Optom. Vis. Sci.*, **69**, 601–608.

Sweeney, D. F. (ed.) (2000) *Silicone Hydrogels: The Rebirth of Continuous Wear Contact Lenses*. Butterworth-Heinemann.

Theodore, F. H. (1963) Superior limbic keratoconjunctivitis. *Ear Nose Throat J.*, **42**, 25–28.

Tomlinson, A. (1992) *Complications of Contact Lens Wear*. Mosby Year Book.

Weber, C. M. and Eichenbaum, J. W. (1997) Acute red eye. Differentiating viral conjunctivitis from other less common causes. *Postgrad. Med.*, **101**, 185–196.

Willcox, M. D. P., Sweeney, D. F., Sharma, S. *et al.* (1995) Culture negative peripheral ulcers are associated with bacterial contamination of contact lenses. *Invest. Ophthalmol. Vis. Sci.*, **36**, S152.

Woods, R. (1989) Quantitative slit lamp observations in contact lens practice. *J. Br. Contact Lens Assoc.*, **12**(Scientific Meetings), 42–45.

Woods, C. A. and Efron, N. (1996) Regular replacement of rigid contact lenses alleviates binding to the cornea. *Int. Contact Lens Clin.*, **23**, 13–18.

Young, G. and Mirejovsky, D. (1993) A hypothesis for the aetiology of soft contact lens-induced superior arcuate keratopathy. *Int. Contact Lens Clin.*, **20**, 177–179.

Zadnik, K. and Mutti, D. O. (1985) Inferior arcuate corneal staining in soft contact lens wearers. *Int. Contact Lens Clin.*, **12**, 110–114.

Zantos, S. G. (1983) Cystic formations in the corneal epithelium during extended wear of contact lenses. *Int. Contact Lens Clin.*, **10**, 128–146.

Zantos, S. G. and Cox, I. (1994) Anterior ocular microscopy – part 1: Biomicroscopy. In *Contact Lens Practice* (M. Ruben and M. Guillon, eds), pp. 359–388, Chapman & Hall.

Zantos, S. G. and Holden, B. A. (1977) Transient endothelial changes soon after wearing soft contact lenses. *Am. J. Optom. Physiol. Opt.*, **54**, 856–858.

2 Microbial keratitis

Barry A. Weissman and Bartly J. Mondino

Introduction

When contact lenses are worn, inconvenience, minor sequelae, and interruptions in wear are commonplace (Herman, 1987). Reversible physiological complications of the anterior ocular structures are not uncommon (Efron, 1999). Corneal complications include superficial punctate staining (Figure 2.1), epithelial microcysts and stromal oedema.

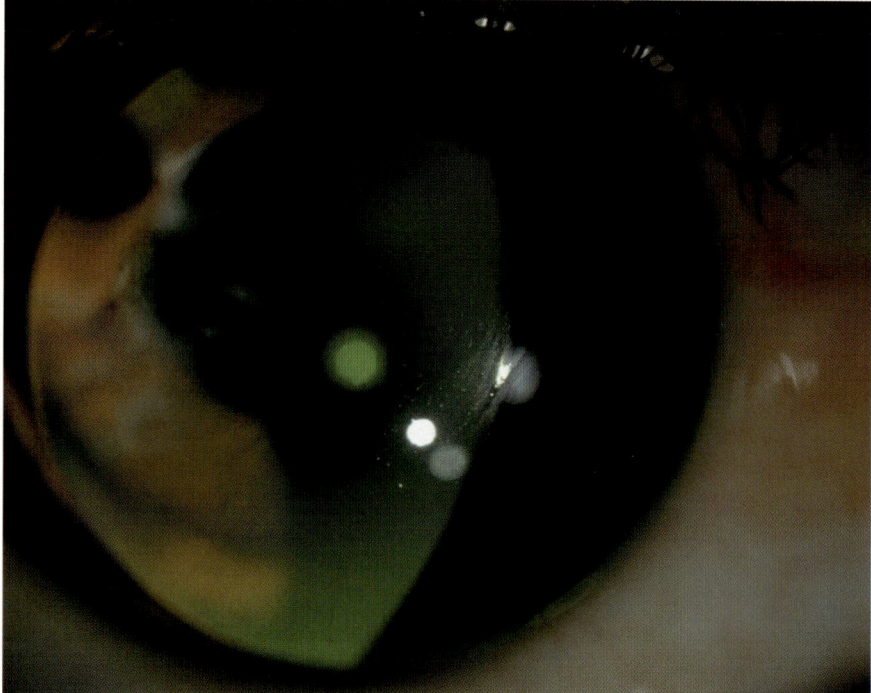

Figure 2.1 Round epithelial abrasion is seen in the aphakic eye of a patient who used a rigid gas-permeable contact lens for daily wear

These may be related to drying, allergic, hypoxic and toxic effects of care solutions; mechanical, contact lens surface or edge problems; or a host of other potential insults. Most of these corneal complications are common but easily treated and managed; they are discussed in detail by Jones and Jones in Chapter 1. Other modest corneal complications, such as abrasions and sterile infiltrates, occur occasionally, but these are usually of short duration and tissue compromise will be limited if wear/care is improved or discontinued.

Contact lenses are known to be potential barriers to corneal oxygen supply (Efron and Ang, 1990). Acute hypoxia induces metabolic changes in the epithelium, resulting in decreased glycogen stores, sensitivity and epithelial adhesion. Epithelial oedema may be clinically observed with the slit lamp as microcysts (Figure 2.2), microcystic

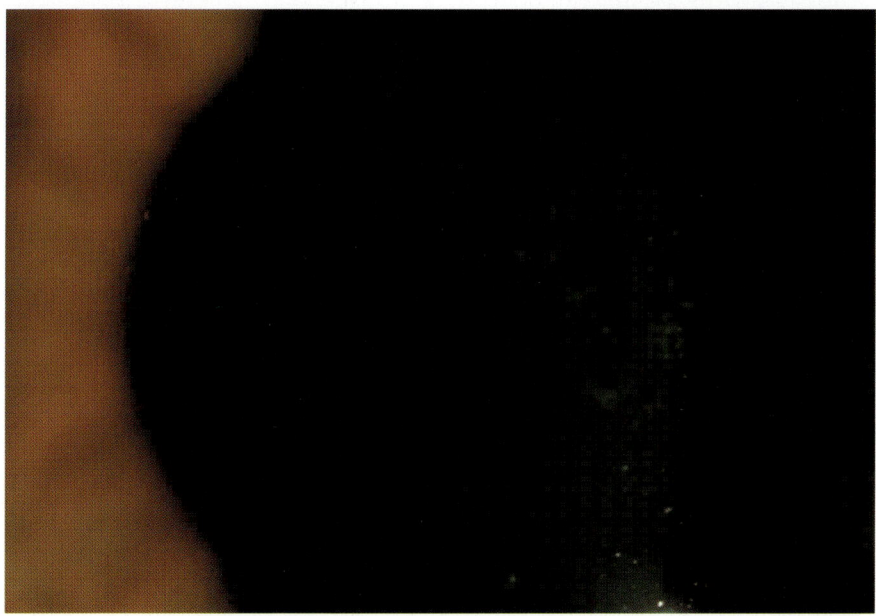

Figure 2.2 Epithelial microcysts seen at the left margin of the pupil in the eye of a patient using hydrogel contact lenses for one week cosmetic extended wear

oedema and oedematous corneal formations. Corneal hypoxia also has been associated with central circular clouding, vascularization of the cornea, acute stromal acidosis and swelling, and chronic stromal thinning, and with changes in endothelial cell morphology (acute blebs and chronic polymegethism) (Efron, 1999). As we advance into a second century of practical contact lens wear, however, contact lens materials and designs that minimize – or even eliminate – corneal hypoxia are now entering the market (Alvord *et al.*, 1998), and concerns about subsequent tissue distress, heretofore of paramount concern, should decline in both prevalence and importance.

The number of patients who suffer severe or permanent compromise of the cornea (restricted to central corneal vascularization (Figure 2.3) or microbial infection and their sequelae) is really quite small (Dixon *et al.*, 1966; Weissman *et al.*, 1987a; Poggio *et al.*, 1989; Rozenman *et al.*, 1989; Schein *et al.*, 1989a; Chan and Weissman, 1996; Shah *et al.*, 1998). The most severe complication of contact lens wear – and a

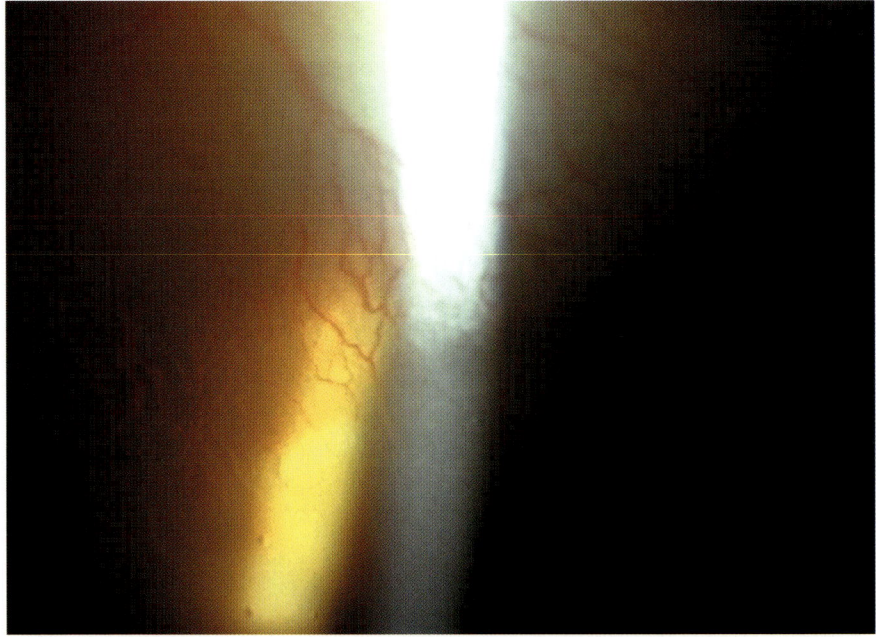

Figure 2.3 Superior corneal pannus following hydrogel contact lens cosmetic extended wear

leading cause of vision loss (Wilhelmus, 1996) through secondary vascularization, scarring, and thinning of the cornea – is direct microbial keratitis. Potential infectious microbes include fungi, viruses and protozoa; however, most corneal infections are associated with bacteria. Fortunately, microbial infection is probably the least commonly encountered complication of contact lens wear.

Pathology and aetiology

The pathophysiology of active corneal infection (ulcerative microbial keratitis) is not yet fully understood, but direct microbial invasion of the intact cornea is relatively rare in healthy individuals. Corneal disease, trauma and surgery, and exposure keratitis (through eyelid disease or disorders of the ocular surface) are well-known factors contributing to microbial infections of the cornea. Contact lens wear has joined this list as a major potential predisposing factor specifically for bacterial corneal infection (and occasionally amoebic or fungal infection as well) during the past two decades (Wilhelmus, 1987). Viral keratitis, particularly herpetic, is a common cause of corneal ulceration, and can become complicated by a secondary bacterial infection; however, this condition has not been specifically associated with contact lens wear and is not the subject of this discussion. In general, the process of infection is believed to depend upon the mechanical, humoral and cellular defence mechanisms of the host on the one hand, and the inoculum size, pathogenicity and virulence of the microorganisms on the other.

Keratitis does not specifically imply an infectious aetiology. Corneal infiltrates are a sign of keratitis (inflammation of the cornea); these are single or multiple transient discrete collections of grey or white material observed in the normally transparent corneal tissues, usually just beneath the epithelium. Infiltrates may be partially or totally inflammatory cells that have migrated through the cornea from the limbal vasculature or from the tears in response to chemotactic factors (cytokines) released from damaged local tissues. Inflammatory cells include polymorphonuclear leucocytes (neutrophils), macrophages and lymphocytes. The small peripheral corneal infiltrates (also called phlyctenules or 'catarrhal' ulcers) associated with *Staphylococcus aureus* blepharitis, for example, tend to be 'sterile', relatively benign and self-limited corneal lesions, specifically representing hypersensitivity to ribitol teichoic acid of the bacterial cell wall (Mondino and Dethlefs, 1984). An infectious agent itself, however, can form all (e.g. in infectious crystalline keratopathy) or part of the infiltrate (Meisler *et al.*, 1984; Reiss *et al.*, 1986; Groden *et al.*, 1987).

Clinical presentation

The typical subjective symptoms of corneal microbial infection are ocular pain, photophobia and decreased vision (with involvement of the corneal visual axis and cells in the anterior chamber). Corneal signs include an epithelial (and perhaps stromal) defect with associated corneal infiltrates and oedema. Both *Acanthamoeba* spp. and *Pseudomonas* spp. infections can result in ring abscesses (note that herpetic keratitis and anaesthetic abuse can mimic this sign). Conjunctival oedema and injection often accompany severe keratitis, as does lid inflammation and an anterior chamber reaction (seen as flare and cells in the aqueous humour). Hypopyon may be associated with severe inflammation of the anterior segment. Mild (or early) keratitis, however, may present with minimal subjective symptoms and clinical signs (Stein *et al.*, 1988).

Both 'sterile' (non-infectious) and infectious corneal infiltrates have been associated with contact lens wear. Mondino and Groden (1980) found that sterile central corneal infiltrates, similar in appearance to those encountered with adenovirus (epidemic keratoconjunctivitis) or chlamydial eye infections, occurred with exposure to contact lens solutions – specifically, ones using thimerosal as a preservative. Similar corneal infiltrates have been associated with contact lenses contaminated with *Streptococcus pneumoniae* (Gordon and Kracher, 1985; Sankaridurg *et al.*, 1999a) and appear to be more common with extended than daily wear of contact lenses (Bates *et al.*, 1989; Donshik *et al.*, 1995; Grant *et al.*, 1998; Holden *et al.*, 1999; Sankaridurg *et al.*, 1999b).

Distinguishing non-infectious sterile infiltrates from active corneal microbial infection is a crucial and often challenging diagnostic step. Stein *et al.* (1988) suggested that active corneal infections were more likely to be associated with increased pain, discharge, epithelial staining, and anterior chamber reaction, whereas sterile infiltrates were usually smaller (most less than 1 mm in diameter), composed of multiple foci, showed minimal superficial punctate epithelial stain, and presented without substantial pain, discharge or anterior chamber reaction. Although central ulcers have been usually considered infectious, Mondino *et al.* (1986), found that 17 of 40 clinically diagnosed corneal infections associated with contact lens wear were peripheral, indicating that the clinician should always have a high index of suspicion irrespective of the location of the affected tissue. Of course, all infections must begin as small infiltrates and/or epithelial defects.

Large studies of corneal infection always include substantial numbers of patients who clinically appear to have microbial keratitis and respond to treatment but who also have had negative culture results for any of numerous reasons (e.g. previous antibiotic therapy, sampling error) (Weissman *et al.*, 1984; Mondino *et al.*, 1986). Considering the risk/benefit of 'overtreating' a sterile infiltrate versus not treating an infectious keratitis, it is probably better to overtreat rather than undertreat any suspicious lesion.

Almost all cases of bacterial corneal ulceration were associated with trauma or concomitant systemic or ocular surface disease until extended-wear contact lenses became popular in the early 1980s. Only 14 cases of 'lost or blinded' eyes, for example, could be documented from a sample of almost 50 000 hard (polymethyl methacrylate, or 'PMMA') contact lens wearers in 1966; eight of these patients were clearly non-compliant with appropriate contact lens care (Dixon *et al.*, 1966). Case reports in the late 1970s suggested an increase in the number of patients presenting with keratitis in parallel with the increasing popularity of hydrogel contact lenses (Freedman and Sugar, 1976; Krachmer and Purcell, 1978). Ruben (1976), on the other hand, concluded from personal clinical experience that the overall incidence of infection with use of hydrogel contact lenses was low – although perhaps somewhat greater than he believed occurred with use of PMMA contact lenses – when hygiene and care were good.

Wilson *et al.* (1981) documented eight corneal ulcers in seven patients using hydrogel contact lenses, and identified the same bacterial serotypes of *Pseudomonas* in the corneal lesions as found in the care systems used by four of seven patients. It is important to note that these patients all used homemade saline inappropriately as a wetting agent, eyedrop or eyebath, following thermal disinfection. This study was the first to link microbial contamination of care solutions with corneal infection.

Cooper and Constable (1977) also reported eight cases of infective keratitis in wearers of hydrogel contact lenses. Four of these eight patients appeared to have no predisposing factors except that they were using contact lenses for 'continuous' or 'extended' wear (one for therapeutic reasons). Three used contact lenses daily or intermittently. The report of Cooper and Constable (1977) thus introduced the modern concern that extended contact lens wear might in some way increase the risk of microbial infection.

It is important to emphasize at this point that the use of all types of contact lenses, including cosmetic (soft, hard, hybrid and gas-permeable) and therapeutic, have been associated with corneal infection at one time or another.

Incidence

Because of difficulties with precise definition, many early reports did not limit their discussions to corneal infection but grouped infectious and non-infectious infiltrates, ulcers and keratitis together. Only active corneal microbial infection occurring in association with contact lens wear should be considered in an analysis of contact lens-induced sight-threatening conditions.

As mentioned above, presentation of corneal infection during cosmetic contact lens wear is a relatively rare event, especially when one restricts observation to daily wear. Even the initial clinical studies of extended wear did not encounter many corneal infections. Only by considering a great panorama of studies over the last 30 years does one come to the inescapable conclusion that something occurs during contact lens extended wear that significantly enhances the risk of this complication.

Salz and Schlanger (1983) presented data on 100 aphakic eyes (70 patients) followed for 3 months to 7 years while using hydrogel contact lenses for extended wear; five corneal 'ulcers' were diagnosed and treated. Eichenbaum et al. (1982) studied another group of 100 aphakic eyes followed for 1 year and found four corneal infections; diabetes was considered a risk factor. Spoor et al. (1984) followed 120 aphakic eyes for 3 years and reported a 4.3% incidence of corneal infection (if all infiltrates are counted, the incidence found by Spoor et al. increases to 6%). These studies were all retrospective clinical studies of solely aphakic eyes using hydrogel contact lenses for extended wear, and report clearly similar results.

Weissman et al. (1987a) discussed a series of corneal infections diagnosed in phakic and aphakic eyes wearing contact lenses for daily and extended wear, treated at a major university hospital (University of California Los Angeles, USA). They concluded that the risk of infection increased some sixfold with extended wear (compared to daily wear), and they did not note any difference in risk between phakic and aphakic eyes. Chalupa et al. (1987) reported a similar experience, observing corneal infection in a large population of contact lens wearers (estimated at 35 000 to 40 000) in Sweden over a 2-year period. They treated and studied 55 corneal infections in these patients during this period, calculating an incidence rate of about 1/15 000 for daily wear and 1/3000 for extended wear of hydrogel lenses.

A large survey of the almost 3000 members of the Contact Lens Section of the American Optometric Association (440 respondees) suggested that corneal infection occurred at an incidence rate of about 0.5% during daily wear and 3% during extended wear of cosmetic hydrogel contact lenses over 2-year blocks of time during the period 1980–1985 (Weissman et al., 1987b).

MacRae et al. (1991) summarized 48 USA Food and Drug Administration (FDA)-controlled studies of new contact lenses between 1980 and 1988, representing the experiences of 22 739 patients. There were 159 serious adverse reactions including 28 'corneal ulcers'. From these data, MacRae et al. (1991) calculated an infection rate of about 1/1500 (events/patient-years) overall for daily wear of contact lenses, 1/244 for cosmetic hydrogel extended wear, and 1/185 for aphakic hydrogel extended wear.

Two important companion studies of corneal infection with both daily and extended cosmetic hydrogel lens wear, sponsored by the USA-based Contact Lens Institute (CLI), were published in the *New England Journal of Medicine* in 1989 (Schein et al., 1989a; Poggio et al., 1989). Use of either daily-wear or extended-wear hydrogel contact lenses under closed eye (extended wear) conditions resulted in a statistically significant increase in risk of infection (9× for daily wear and 10–15× for extended wear). Moreover, the risk of infection appeared to increase with each additional night of wear. The annualized incidence of corneal infection was 21/10 000 for extended wear and 4/10 000 for daily wear (Schein *et al.*, 1989a; Poggio *et al.*, 1989). These data were confirmed in a European study a decade later (Cheung *et al.*, 1999).

Summarizing the above, while the risk of infection in patients using the contact lenses available in the 1980s was really quite low, this risk clearly increased during extended wear. The incidence of infection with cosmetic daily-wear lenses appeared to be about 0.1% per year. Cosmetic extended wear may increase this incidence to about 0.5–1% per year, whereas aphakic extended wear is potentially more hazardous at almost 2% per year.

Ocular defence factors

The blinking action of the lid and the flow of tears over the anterior segment of the eye mechanically removes microorganisms. Tears are relatively cool and nutrient poor, and contain various antibacterial substances, such as lysozyme, betalysin, lactoferrin and mucus (which envelops microorganisms). Tears also contain secretory IgA, as well as the alternative pathway of complement factors, which can trap and coat microorganisms, suppress adhesion and alter binding to the surface antigens of microbes – all of which can enhance lysis and phagocytosis.

The corneal epithelium poses a formidable mechanical barrier to most microbes. Only *Corynebacterium diphtheriae*, *Listeria* spp., *Neisseria gonorrhoeae*, and *Haemophilus aegyptius* (Koch–Weeks bacillus) are believed able to invade the intact corneal epithelium (Jones, 1978; Ogawa and Hyndiuk, 1994).

It is felt that the normal ocular microbial flora of the conjunctiva and ocular adnexa exist in a stable balance between proliferation and control by the various indigenous antibacterial factors discussed above. Staphylococci and diphtheroids predominated in ocular cultures from 10 271 individuals aged 1 to 90 years (Locatcher-Khorazo *et al.*, 1972b). The normal bacteria are thought to protect the tissues from colonization by organisms of greater virulence and pathogenic potential.

Risk factors

The ocular defence mechanisms described above are constantly being challenged by a variety of specific risk factors that are believed to encourage the infectious process during contact lens use.

Extended wear

'Extended wear' implies that contact lens wear is 'extended' through one or multiple sleep cycles before cleaning and 'disinfection'. This concept should be distinguished from 'continuous' wear, which implies that contact lenses are never removed for routine cleaning. Non-compliant patients (as opposed to clinicians) probably introduced cosmetic extended wear. Anecdotal reports of rare patients 'safely' napping or sleeping with PMMA contact lenses still on the eye, perhaps 'parked' on the sclera, were common 30 and 40 years ago.

Soon after hydrogel contact lenses were introduced, these devices were prescribed as continuous-wear bandages to treat diseases of the ocular surface. Complications were common but disasters few. Dohlman *et al.* (1973) found that 11 of 278 bandage hydrogel contact lens patients developed corneal infiltrates. Four patients suffered definite microbial infections, resulting in permanent damage to the eyes. These authors concluded, however, that the advantages of therapeutic continuous contact lens wear in the treatment of eye disease far outweighed the risks.

The 'Permalens' was developed in about 1970 by DeCarle, working in the UK. This was perhaps the first hydrogel contact lens design intended for extended wear, and was originally fitted using a very small diameter and steep back central curvature, compared to other hydrogel contact lenses of the day. In June 1979, the US Food and Drug Administration (FDA) approved the use of two extended-wear hydrogel contact lens designs – Permalens and Hydrocurve – initially to be prescribed only for aphakia (Hartstein, 1982).

Early clinical reports of the US experience suggested that extended wear was successful and safe (Stark *et al.*, 1979; Binder and Woodward, 1980; Stark and Martin, 1981); complications occurred, but the risks appeared similar to those encountered with daily wear. The benefit of patient convenience led to much satisfaction among both phakic and aphakic patients, perhaps justifying the anticipated limited risk.

Another clinical trial in the UK also concluded that continual wear (only for 20 weeks) of Sauflon 85 hydrogel contact lenses was innocuous (for only 20 subjects). Although several indices of corneal integrity were monitored, only a decrease in corneal sensitivity and perhaps central stromal thickness, and an increase in contact lens soilage, were noted (Hirji and Larke, 1979; Larke and Hirji, 1979).

The report of Cooper and Constable (1977) from Perth, Australia (see above) was perhaps the first warning of a problem. Zantos and Holden (1978), also in Australia, originally intended to enrol 100 patients to wear a variety of contact lenses for continuous wear for up to 2 years. They observed multiple complications, however, including corneal oedema, neovascularization, microcysts, 12 instances of acute red eye reactions, and several infections. Three patients developed small marginal ulcers and one presented with multiple small central epithelial lesions, which later coalesced into a large central ulcer. Every patient who attempted continuous wear experienced some difficulty resulting in an interruption of wear, and the study was terminated after the first 35 patients.

As extended wear proliferated throughout North America in the early 1980s, the original glowing reports faded and the reality predicted by the Australian observations became clear. Several reports in the early 1980s provided evidence that extended wear was associated with a higher rate of corneal infection in both aphakic and phakic patients. Mondino *et al.* (1986), for example, studied 40 patients who presented with corneal infections associated with contact lens wear. Eleven of these patients wore lenses solely for daily wear, and all were found to be non-compliant with appropriate care (e.g. eight patients reported occasionally sleeping with their lenses on their eyes!). Twenty-nine patients used FDA extended-wear approved hydrogel contact lenses for extended wear (for 3 days to 30 months). Twelve were found to be compliant with the then-current care guidelines, and of the non-compliant 17, the most common defect in compliance was microbial contamination of care systems. This study highlights the conclusion that must be reached from the literature reviewed above: specific risk factors for corneal infection during contact lens wear include: (1) extended wear, and (2) non-compliance with contact lens care procedures and hygiene. As perhaps 70 million people worldwide now wear contact lenses, often for extended wear, it is not surprising that many believe that contact lens-related microbial keratitis has the potential of becoming an important public health concern.

Hypoxia

Oxygen tension (expressed in torr or mmHg) is found by multiplying the percentage of oxygen in the air by the barometric pressure (the presence of water vapour introduces only slight errors into this calculation). As oxygen accounts for about 21% of the atmosphere and sea-level pressure is given as 760 mmHg, normal sea-level oxygen tension is about 155 mmHg. Polse and Mandell (1970) proposed that there was an anterior corneal 'critical oxygen tension' (COT), below which corneal metabolism would be compromised. By use of a goggle through which gases of specified oxygen concentrations were passed, and observation of sub-sequent corneal swelling, these authors suggested that the COT was 11–19 mmHg. The COT criterion of Polse and Mandell (1970) represents about 2% of the oxygen tension at sea level. Later human goggle studies, with better controls and additional subjects, showed that the COT to prevent corneal oedema should be more like 40–70 mmHg (5–10% O_2) (Mandell and Farrell, 1970; Holden *et al.*, 1984).

Holden and Mertz (1984) used contact lenses of known oxygen transmissibilities (Dk/t) (on a limited number of subjects) to determine the 'critical Dk/t'. They suggested that human corneal swelling could be precluded by use of contact lenses with Dk/t values of 24×10^{-9} (cm/s)$\times$(mlO_2/ml$\times$mmHg) for daily wear conditions or 87×10^{-9} (cm/s)$\times$(mlO_2/ml$\times$mmHg) for extended wear. Either of these situations presumably permits an oxygen tension of 40–70 mmHg or more under contact lenses. Few hydrogel contact lenses available through the 1980s met even their daily wear criterion, and only recently (Alvord et al., 1998) have contact lenses been developed that come close to the Holden–Mertz extended-wear critical Dk/t value. It is also valuable to note that both human corneal oxygen utilization (Larke et al., 1981) and oxygenation of the palpebral conjunctiva (Efron and Carney, 1979; Isenberg and Green, 1985) vary substantially from individual to individual, limiting the usefulness of such criteria for specific patients.

It has been proposed that hypoxia at the corneal surface results in metabolic compromise of the epithelium, which renders the epithelium less resistant to microbial infection (Imayasu et al., 1994). Although hypoxia causes numerous metabolic problems for the cornea – resulting in multiple changes in the epithelium, stroma and endothelium – the link between these problems and microbial keratitis has yet to be established. It is also clear, however, that all extended-wear hydrogel contact lenses, used on a wearing schedule ranging from 4 to 28 nights in a row, cause ocular complications. In one study, no severe infections were encountered, but superficial punctate epithelial staining, epithelial microcysts, red eye reactions and other changes occurred at similar rates across several wearing schedules (Kenyon et al., 1986).

Non-compliance

Another identified risk factor is that of non-compliance with contact lens care techniques (Claydon and Efron, 1994). Mondino et al. (1986) provided a definition of compliance with contact lens wear. A compliant patient washes hands before any contact lens manipulations, appropriately uses an FDA-approved care system in a manner in agreement with both the published guidelines of the manufacturer and good hygiene, adheres to the recommended wear schedule (for either daily or extended wear), and is found to have no microbial contamination of solutions and cases.

Wilson et al. (1981) established the link between poor contact lens care and hygiene and corneal infection by demonstrating the same serotype of Pseudomonas in corneal ulcers and the care systems of their patients. Garwood (1991) presented data suggesting that corneal infection incidence increases more than 10-fold when cleaning and disinfection techniques are not employed with daily wear use of hydrogel contact lenses.

Both Collins and Carney (1986) and Chun and Weissman (1987) studied compliance and found that 40–70% of contact lens users were non-compliant by history. Claydon *et al.* (1997) failed in their attempt to enhance compliance by subjecting patients to a more thorough initial instruction protocol concerning contact lens wear and care procedures, which emphasizes the importance of developing other strategies to enhance patient compliance.

Several authors have studied microbial contamination of contact lens solutions and cases. Pitts and Krachmer (1979) cultured the cases and conjunctivae of 29 patients and found that 10 (34%) had contaminated cases despite use of heat disinfection. Donzis *et al.* (1987) cultured all elements of the care systems of 100 asymptomatic contact lens users, including 38 rigid contact lens users and 62 hydrogel contact lens users (50 daily wear and 12 extended wear). More than 50% of these patients had microbial contamination in some element of their care system; the microbes found by culture included potential pathogenic bacteria such as Gram-negative *Pseudomonas* and *Serratia*, Gram-positive *Staphylococcus* and *Bacillus*, as well as two cultures positive for the protozoan *Acanthamoeba*.

Campbell and Caroline (1990) suggested that even patients who use care regimens compliantly may not be able to avoid microbial contamination of their care systems. They suggest that care systems that are effective during manufacturer studies may later become ineffective in the home environment because the bacteria encountered are more resistant through development of bacterial biofilm. Thirty-nine of 45 patients studied used their disinfection techniques correctly, yet 29% of their patients using heat disinfection, 50% using peroxide disinfection, and 75% of those using chemical disinfection, provided cases from which bacteria were recovered.

Microbes adhere to contact lens surfaces, most likely by formation of biofilms. The contact lens may then act as a vector, transferring pathogenic agents from the contaminated case and/or solutions directly to the ocular surface. As *Pseudomonas* appears to be responsible for 50–70% of culture-positive corneal infections in contact lens wearers (see below), the ability of several subtypes of this particular microorganism to attach to corneas as well as to all forms of contact lenses (new and worn, rigid and hydrogel, high and low water content, ionic and non-ionic) has been studied. However, the exact role of bacterial adherence in the pathogenesis of corneal infection has yet to be clearly described (Baum and Panjwani, 1988). It seems unlikely that bacteria trapped in a biofilm on a contact lens surface could infect an eye, but their progeny might do so.

The source of these microbes is still unclear. Schein *et al.* (1989b) specifically point out that the relative paucity of corneal infections involving enteric bacteria (such as *E. coli*, *Proteus* and *Klebsiella*) argues against faecal contamination. Bacteria cultured from 'healthy' (non-contact lens-wearing) eyes are those commonly found also on the skin and in the upper respiratory tract (i.e. staphylococci and diphtheroids), and these have indeed been associated with some contact lens-associated corneal infections. Moreover, wet areas in the bathroom and kitchen, such as taps (faucets) and sinks, are often contaminated with Gram-negative bacteria (specifically *Pseudomonas*). Wilcox *et al.* (1997) presented data suggesting that Gram-negative bacteria are indeed derived from the domestic water supply, whereas other bacteria most likely have the lid margins as their source. Acanthamoeba is ubiquitous.

Blepharitis

Patients presenting for initial or continued contact lens care who show signs of blepharitis or dacryocystis are believed to be at greater risk of infection because there is a known source of pathogenic microbes in close proximity to the ocular surface.

Signs of acute blepharitis include inflammation of the lid margins, flaky debris on the eyelashes, and yellow or frothy exudates. Chronic blepharitis is often associated with meibomian gland dysfunction and blockage, telangiectatic and dilated blood vessels, and perhaps small irregularities (notches) in the lid margin. The bulbar conjunctiva may be either white or inflamed, and the cornea may be clear or may exhibit superficial staining, especially inferiorly. Some patients suffer from recurrent styes and chalazia, or hordeoli.

The tear film is often compromised in blepharitis. Debris is noted in the tear fluid, and tear film breakup time is abnormally short. This is partially due to interference with the normal production of sebum from the meibomian glands, and the rain of bacterial toxins and metabolic waste products falling into the palpebral aperture. Mechanical irregularities in the apposition of the diseased lid margins to the globe may further compromise the tears.

Patients commonly present to ophthalmic practices with small, marginal limbal 'sterile ulcers' or phlyctenules. Although corneal phlyctenules and peripheral infiltrates may initially be sterile, it is presumed that any epithelial defect increases the risk of a secondary direct infection, especially when bandaged by a contact lens and considering the proximity of available microbes.

Staphylococcus spp. are known to be important agents in blepharitis, but many other microbes may be involved, including other bacteria and even arthropods such as lice or the follicle mite *Demodex folliculorum*.

Patients who suffer from acne rosacea are particularly at risk for blepharitis (usually associated with *S. aureus*), corneal neovascularization and corneal ulceration/infection even when no contact lenses are worn.

Diabetes mellitus

Diabetes mellitus has been suggested as a risk factor for corneal infection, specifically when contact lenses are used for extended wear. Eichenbaum *et al.* (1982) studied 100 aphakic patients who wore hydrogel contact lenses on an extended-wear basis, and all three patients who were diabetic developed infections. A fourth patient, who concomitantly had cancer of the colon, also developed a corneal infection. None of 135 control patients wearing spectacles (eight diabetics) developed corneal infections. Spoor *et al.* (1984) found that their data supported this conclusion.

Diabetic patients have systemic metabolic abnormalities that theoretically place them at greater risk for microbial infections. O'Leary and Millodot (1981) determined that both contact lens wear and diabetes specifically result in abnormal fragility of the corneal epithelial layer. However, O'Donnell *et al.* (2001) were unable to find any evidence of significant ocular compromise in a prospective, randomized, masked, controlled experiment that followed the progress of 40 diabetic contact lens wearers versus 40 non-diabetic contact lens wearers for 12 months.

Other forms of immunosuppression may also increase the risk of acquiring corneal infection during contact lens wear, or potentiate the severity of the disease should it occur.

Epithelial trauma

Epithelial trauma while wearing, removing or inserting a contact lens possibly plays a role in subsequent corneal infection. As noted above, the intact corneal epithelium presents a substantial barrier to infection. Before a microbe can establish an infection, it must adhere to its target. Experimental bacterial inoculation of linear abrasions has been effective in first increasing adherence of *Pseudomonas aeruginosa* to the corneal tissues and then producing corneal ulceration (Ramphal *et al.*, 1981; Hyndiuk, 1981; Stern *et al.*, 1985). Stern *et al.* (1982) showed that *Pseudomonas* adheres better to injured or exposed basal epithelial cells than to an intact epithelial surface or even to exposed bare corneal stroma.

Adams *et al.* (1983) found that five of six patients presenting with corneal infections associated with extended wear of hydrogel contact lenses reported recent manipulations of their contact lenses. These authors speculated that this might have led to epithelial defects that predisposed these patients to the infectious process. Mondino *et al.* (1986), however, could not support this particular hypothesis with data from their patient group.

Minor epithelial erosions are commonly seen in all contact lens wearers (Weissman *et al.*, 1994). What is not clear, however, is why such lesions appear to be relatively innocuous when contact lenses are used on a daily-wear basis, and if, or how, the role of such lesions changes during extended wear. Some believe that treatment of minor epithelial staining with prophylactic topical antibiotics represents cautious practice, whereas others feel that this practice risks encouraging resistance among local bacteria and hence eventual 'superinfection', and that the toxicity of some antibiotics may actually prolong the healing process.

Direct damage may not be necessary to initiate the infectious process in the cornea during contact lens wear. An electron microscopy study of primate corneal epithelia after use of excessively thick hydrogels for daily or extended wear showed epithelial thinning (loss of superficial cells and flattening of the remaining ones), oedema, and degenerative cytoplasmic changes (Bergmanson *et al.*, 1985) (see Chapter 4). Imayasu *et al.* (1994) reported that contact lens-induced hypoxia increases the binding of *Pseudomonas* to corneal epithelial cells.

Steroid use

Topical corticosteroid use is generally recognized as an exacerbating factor with corneal microbial infection (Dohlman *et al.*, 1973; Jones, 1981), particularly infections involving herpes, *Pseudomonas* spp. and fungi. Steroids suppress immunological defence mechanisms and inflammatory reactions (as well as increasing the risks of glaucoma and cataract formation), and by doing so may also mask the severity of an infection. Chalupa *et al.* (1987) identified inappropriate steroid therapy as a major factor contributing to the severity of corneal infection after contact lens wear.

Therapeutic/bandage contact lens use

Therapeutic contact lenses are occasionally employed to protect the corneal surface, facilitate healing and relieve pain in patients suffering from filamentary keratitis, bullous keratopathy, persistent non-healing epithelial defects (including those found following refractive surgery procedures), exposed sutures (e.g. after keratoplasty), neurotrophic or exposure keratitis, keratitis sicca and ocular pemphigoid. All of these situations involve disruption of the epithelial surface barrier. Many patients suffering from these conditions are elderly, some are diabetic, and often they are using topical corticosteroids. The combination of known risk factors is believed to place these patients at particular risk, and it is not surprising that infection is a major concern in this group (Dohlman *et al.*, 1973; Kent *et al.*, 1990).

As an example of the above concerns, six corneal ulcers (both bacterial and fungal by culture) developed in 38 eyes treated with therapeutic hydrogel contact lenses for severe epithelial diseases including Stevens–Johnson and Sjögren syndromes, ocular pemphigoid, neurotrophic keratitis, herpes simplex keratitis, and ocular burns (Brown *et al.*, 1974). Several factors were felt to contribute to these infections, including concurrent dry eye, use of antibiotics and steroids, and microbial contamination of a bottle of sodium chloride drops in one case.

Tobacco use

In studies of corneal infection associated with contact lens wear by the Contact Lens Institute (Schein *et al.*, 1989a; Poggio *et al.*, 1989), a number of potential risk factors were investigated, including age, sex and race of patients, the age of the contact lens and type of fit (initial or replacement), length of time since last professional evaluation, and identification of providing professional. The only factor of these that appeared to have some statistical relation to corneal infection was smoking, which was statistically significant for extended-wear use of contact lenses and almost significant for daily wear as well. Data from Cutter *et al.* (1996) supported this observation with regard to the occurrence of non-infectious corneal infiltrates in association with hydrogel contact lens wear. The mechanism by which tobacco use renders the cornea of contact lens wearers more susceptible to infection remains unclear.

Other potential risk factors

Some clinical reports have suggested additional risk factors for the development of microbial keratitis among contact lens wearers, such as travel and warm weather (Donzis, 1998), but these have not been scientifically verified.

Microorganisms

Some forms of the microorganisms among which we all live are symbiotic, aiding us in such processes as the digestion of our food and producing vitamins as byproducts of their own metabolism. Others ignore human life, and appear to remain invisible to our existence. Some microbes are well known as human pathogens; many more do not usually cause difficulties but are capable of inducing human disease if given the appropriate opportunity. Studies of the normal flora of the ocular surface suggest a predominance of staphylococci and diphtheroids (Locatcher-Khorazo et al., 1972b). Species of greater potential virulence are only rarely encountered.

Neisser was perhaps the first to isolate and describe a microbial ocular pathogen, the gonococcus, in 1879. Koch observed the second such microbe while studying the aetiology of cholera in Egypt, and Weeks later isolated this bacterium, now known as the Koch–Weeks bacillus, or *Haemophilus aegypticus*. *Streptococcus pneumoniae* was first identified as a common cause of central corneal infections in 1893. Morax isolated a diplobacillus from a case of subacute angular conjunctivitis in 1897; this bacterium was independently identified by Axenfeld and is known as *Moraxella lacunata* (Gasparrini, 1893; Locatcher-Khorazo et al., 1972a).

Many potential corneal microbial pathogens have since been identified and those now particularly associated with corneal infection after contact lens wear are discussed below.

Bacteria

Bacteria have been classically grouped according to their morphology (rod, spiral or coccus), their reaction to Gram, Giemsa or other stains, and other aspects of their biochemistry (e.g. coagulase-negative, fastidious nutrition). Modern microbiology has only recently begun to reorganize its taxonomy around information retrieved from molecular biology.

The clinician cannot make a specific and reliable aetiological diagnosis based solely on the clinical appearance of a corneal ulcer. Corneal ulcers associated with Gram-positive bacteria, however, tend to be smaller, more localized and distinct, and relatively less purulent and aggressive, compared with those associated with Gram-negative bacteria. With no or improper therapy, perforation may occur within several days, even when Gram-positive bacteria are involved.

Gram-positive bacteria

Both *Staphylococcus epidermidis* and *S. aureus* are very common Gram-positive inhabitants of normal human skin, particularly the eyelid. *S. aureus* causes a wide variety of pyogenic (pus-forming) infections and is a common cause of food poisoning. *S. aureus* is also well established as a cause of both conjunctivitis and blepharitis and has been associated with corneal marginal infiltrates and phlyctenules. Both *Staphylococcus* species have also been frequently cultured from corneal infections, both with and without contact lens wear.

Streptococcus pneumoniae and *S. pyogenes* are two other Gram-positive bacteria commonly cultured from corneal ulcers. *S. pneumoniae* (the pneumococcus), in particular, exists as part of the normal human adult flora of the upper respiratory tract, where it can be a reservoir for both pneumonia as well as ear and eye infections. *Streptococcus* spp. commonly produce hypopyon and are felt to be more aggressive in the cornea than *S. aureus*, which is, in turn, more aggressive than *S. epidermidis*. Under certain conditions (e.g. topical steroid treatment) certain bacteria (especially *Streptococcus viridans*, another common normal inhabitant of the upper respiratory tract) may multiply under an intact epithelium to assume an arborizing crystalline appearance (Meisler *et al.*, 1984; Reiss *et al.*, 1986; Groden *et al.*, 1987).

A study of more than 3500 corneal ulcer cultures (from 1938 to 1968) in New York suggested that 85% were associated with either *Staphylococcus* or *Streptococcus* species; only 194 positive cultures of *P. aeruginosa* were found (Locatcher-Khorazo *et al.*, 1972a).

Another Gram-positive bacterium, *Bacillus* spp., occasionally causes both corneal infection and severe endophthalmitis (*B. cereus*, in particular, has emerged as a potentially virulent intraocular pathogen) (Ormerod and Smith, 1986; Donzis *et al.*, 1988). *Bacillus* spp. have been found in the contact lens care systems of about 5% of asymptomatic patients (Donzis *et al.*, 1987); these bacteria form spores that are resistant to heat and to many forms of chemical disinfectants. Heat treatement of 121°C for 15 minutes, or 5 hours of exposure to 3% hydrogen peroxide, however, should eliminate viable forms of this bacteria (Donzis *et al.*, 1988).

Gram-negative bacteria

Pseudomonas spp. (principally *aeruginosa*) are Gram-negative, slender, rod-shaped bacteria capable of producing devastating corneal infections. *Pseudomonas* is a ubiquitous microorganism in nature, distributed widely in soil, water, plants, the mammalian gut, and in sewage. In the home, *P. aeruginosa* is often found in and around sinks and other wet areas. It can utilize many different organic compounds (including atmospheric carbon dioxide) as a source of carbon and energy, and is able to contaminate fluorescein solutions, eye cosmetics, saline and distilled water. *Pseudomonas* rarely causes systemic infections in healthy individuals but can become a major pathogen when the opportunity presents, causing pneumonia in myelosuppressed cancer patients and sepsis after burns. It is a common cause of death in victims of cystic fibrosis.

It has been thought that *Pseudomonas* spp. are not able to invade the intact corneal epithelium but aggressively destroy corneal tissues once a wound has allowed adhesion by a sufficient load of these bacteria (Hyndiuk, 1981; Stern *et al.*, 1982, 1985). Recent research contests this view, suggesting that at least some strains are more 'toxic' than others and can invade intact epithelium (Fleiszig *et al.*, 1998). *Pseudomonas* liberates endotoxins, exotoxins and proteolytic enzymes (proteases) and can thus lead to a rapidly progressive corneal ulcer characterized by melting and purulence. Patients with *Pseudomonas* corneal infections often present with large epithelial defects, dense anterior stromal infiltrates, severe stromal oedema, and mucoid material clinging to the lesion. Ring infiltrates may be seen. The host immunoreaction to the stromal infection may be partially responsible for the rapid, massive and persistent destruction of corneal structure in this disease.

Serratia marcescens is another Gram-negative rod also capable of liberating endotoxin, but corneal infections are generally not quite as severe as those associated with *Pseudomonas*. *Serratia* can develop resistance to certain preservatives often used in contact lens care systems, such as benzalkonium chloride and chlorhexidine.

The endotoxin released by Gram-negative bacteria such as *Pseudomonas* and *Serratia* is heat resistant and may therefore not be eliminated from contact lens care systems even after thermal disinfection has killed all bacteria. Endotoxin is itself immunogenic and, even in the absence of viable bacteria, has been shown to cause corneal ring infiltrates (Belmont *et al.*, 1982).

Moraxella spp. (Gram-negative diplobacilli; principally *M. lacunata*) are well known as ocular pathogens, especially in angular blepharitis. They are usually associated with corneal infection in debilitated individuals such as chronic alcoholics, and have only occasionally been identified in corneal infection associated with contact lens wear.

Other bacteria

Although the usual bacterial pathogens detailed above are well known and are recovered from the vast majority of corneal infections, the clinician must always be on guard for the rare contaminant. Several other bacteria have occasionally been cultured from both contact lens care systems and infected corneas of contact lens wearers. *Propionibacterium acnes* is an example of a Gram-positive bacterium occasionally cultured from corneal infections after contact lens wear. Similarly, Gram-negative organisms occasionally found by culture include the enteric bacteria *Klebsiella* and *Proteus*. Corneal lesions also give mixed or even negative culture results.

Fungi

Although fungal deposits in hydrogel contact lens have been reported by several authors, corneal infection has been very rare. Wilson and Ahearn (1986) reported 11 instances of fungal contact lens contamination from 450 patients using hydrogel contact lenses (extended wear) during a clinical experience of 5 years. These authors found only two instances of associated corneal fungal infection, but the same organism was found in the contact lens growths and eye lesions in both these events. One fungus was *Fusarium verticilloides* and the other *Curvularia lunata*. Several additional patients experienced ocular injection, corneal staining and irritation while wearing these contaminated contact lenses, and the authors felt it likely that liberated fungal toxins were involved. Other fungi commonly identified in human corneal ulcers, but not specific to contact lens wear, are *Candida* (a yeast) and *Aspergillus*. Penley *et al.* (1985) suggested that either heat disinfection or at least 45 minutes of soaking in 3% hydrogen peroxide would eliminate viable fungi from contaminated hydrogel contact lenses.

Fungal ulcers can clinically appear chronic and indolent or acute and severe, depending on the exact organism and the host status. They are often difficult to diagnose as initial cultures are frequently negative. Biopsy can be helpful. Fungal corneal infections may demonstrate feathery borders (hyphate edges), raised infiltrates, endothelial plaque, and 'satellite' lesions on slit lamp examination.

Viruses

Both herpetic and adenoviral corneal infections are commonly diagnosed and treated in ophthalmic practice. Herpetic corneal infection is considered a major cause of blindness. Herpes simplex is known as the 'great imitator' of corneal infection and should be considered in the differential diagnosis of most corneal diseases, especially when a dendritic lesion and/or a loss of corneal sensitivity are present. Corneal disease related to adenoviral infection, whether explosive epidemic keratoconjunctivitis or milder varieties, is self-limiting. Although transient subepithelial infiltrates and punctate subepithelial scars are common sequelae, this infection rarely leads to severe permanent visual loss. Both of these viral infections, and others like Thygeson's keratitis (Figure 2.4), are occasionally encountered in patients concomitantly wearing contact lenses, and could be spread through poor care of diagnostic contact lenses.

The human immunodeficiency virus (HIV) has been isolated from the tears, conjunctiva and corneas of infected individuals (Fujikawa *et al.*, 1986) but there have been no documented cases suggesting that this disease can be transmitted through any form of ocular contact or contact

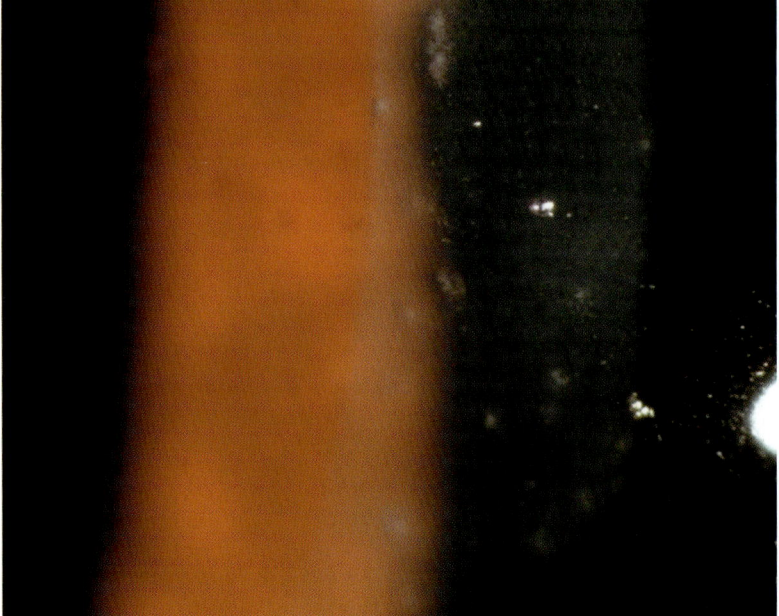

Figure 2.4 Epithelial infiltrates seen in a patient suffering from Thygeson's keratitis

lens wear. Nevertheless, it is essential (and indeed mandatory in the USA) to disinfect all office instruments and diagnostic contact lenses between patients (and in the USA to follow Center for Disease Control guidelines for all patient care activities).

It is intuitive, moreover, that patients suffering from HIV infection, as well as other immunodeficient states, are at some increased risk for microbial keratitis while wearing contact lenses, and if such infection develops, both the initiation of the disease and its course may be potentiated by immune system compromise (Nanda *et al.*, 1991).

Protozoa

Acanthamoebas are a group of free-living protozoa found ubiquitously in soil, water and air across a broad range of climatic and environmental conditions. They exist in two forms – mobile trophozoites and cysts – the latter of which has a double wall and therefore contributes to the impressive resistance of this microorganism.

Corneal infection associated with *Acanthamoeba* was first reported by Naginton in 1974. Although only a small number had been reported until

1981, a dramatic increase was seen in the mid–1980s, particularly among contact lens users. The observation that *Acanthamoeba* keratitis occurs in patients who had previously healthy eyes but used homemade saline as part of their contact lens care was made by Moore *et al.* (1985).

Infection has been attributed to exposure to non-sterile water sources during contact lens use or swimming, including tapwater, well water, water from a home 'purification kit', saline intended for intravenous use, and even saliva, although such assertions have recently been contested (Chynn *et al.*, 1997). Daily wear of hydrogel contact lenses appears to be the primary predisposing mode of contact lens use, but several other types of contact lens wear have also been associated with this infection, including extended wear of hydrogel, rigid and rigid-hydrogel hybrid ('Saturn') contact lenses (Koenig *et al.*, 1987; Moore *et al.*, 1987).

Stehr-Green *et al.* (1988) reviewed the epidemiology of more than a decade of *Acanthamoeba* keratitis in the USA. These authors studied 208 case reports, of which 189 provided information regarding suspected risk factors. Contact lenses of many types were worn by 85% of these patients, and 64% of the wearers had a history of use of salt tablet-prepared saline. They suggest that merely rinsing a rigid gas-permeable lens in tapwater prior to ocular insertion is a risk factor for this disease. In this series, however, patients aged 50 years and above commonly had a concomitant history of ocular trauma.

The clinical features of *Acanthamoeba* infection include a long progressive history of severe pain and photophobia, central or paracentral infiltrates (early in the disease course; see Figure 2.5), and ring infiltrates (similar in clinical appearance to the ring infiltrates seen in *P. aeruginosa* infection) late in the disease course. Additional signs include a dendriform epithelial lesion (often clinically suggestive of herpetic keratitis), recurrent epithelial breakdown, radial keratoneuritis and chemosis. There is usually an anterior chamber reaction, and occasionally sclerokeratitis. Initial cultures and smears are often negative unless special techniques (i.e. calcofluor white stain or culturing on non-nutrient agar with an *E. coli* overlay) and deeper biopsy are used.

Management

Management of corneal infection with contact lens wear includes prevention, rapid diagnosis and appropriate treatment.

Prevention

The two principal risk factors identified for corneal infection associated with cosmetic contact lens wear are believed to be extended wear and

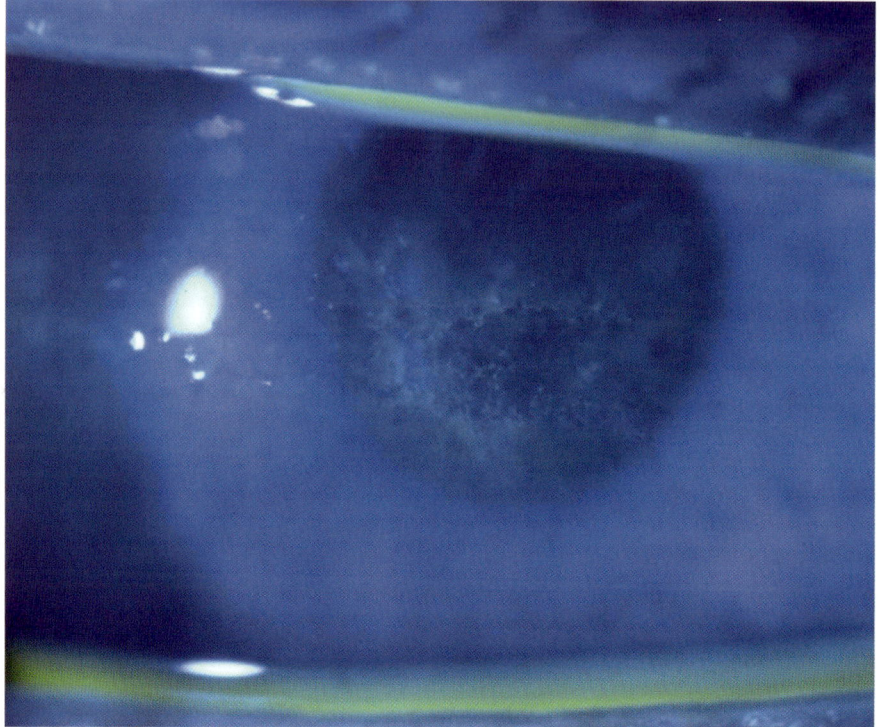

Figure 2.5 Epithelial changes in an early *Acanthamoeba* keratitis associated with contact lens wear

inappropriate care techniques. The therapeutic use of hydrogel contact lenses is considered a third major risk factor, but this risk is often unavoidable and the benefits are thought to outweigh the risks.

Prevention consists of minimizing the risk to patients by avoiding the use of contact lenses for extended wear as much as possible. In cases where such use is necessary (e.g. sometimes in the management of paediatric aphakia or the use of hydrogel contact lenses as bandages), patients (or their guardians) should provide informed consent and, being alerted to these risks, should present without delay if any signs or symptoms of infection occur. Even in the dawn of 'super' oxygen-permeable silicone hydrogel lenses, cosmetic extended wear should be approached with caution.

Important measures in decreasing the risk of infection (particularly by *Acanthamoeba*) include compliant and hygienic use of contact lens care regimens, elimination of the use of 'homemade' saline solutions, and minimizing exposure to non-sterile water. In the case of swimming, the risk of infection can be reduced by wearing airtight goggles over the lenses, or removing lenses immediately after swimming with contact lenses on the eyes; or avoided by adopting the more stringent precaution of not wearing contact lenses at all while swimming.

Contact lens wear should be discontinued during illness (colds and flu), episodes of ocular irritation, and in the presence of ipsilateral or contralateral ocular or adnexal microbial infection.

Yet a third additional preventive measure is routine professional care and supervision. Contact lens patients should obtain professional evaluations at scheduled intervals of perhaps 6–9 months under normal conditions, but more frequently (e.g. perhaps every 2–4 months) if any increased risk is suspected. This could include instances of therapeutic use, following corneal grafts, and in patients who smoke and/or wear lenses on an extended-wear basis.

Immunosuppressed or diabetic patients, and patients who present with severely compromised tear films, acne rosacea, chronic blepharitis, overtly poor personal hygiene, or use of topical ophthalmic steroids (e.g. to control uveitis) should probably be discouraged from cosmetic contact lens wear; if contact lenses must be worn for cosmesis or some other benefit (e.g. aphakia), use should be restricted to daily wear if at all possible.

Early recognition and diagnosis

Patients must participate actively in their own care. Every contact lens wearer, particularly those using extended wear on occasion or regularly, should know the signs and symptoms of corneal infection:

- ocular pain and/or photophobia;
- conjunctival injection;
- lid oedema;
- tearing;
- possibly discharge or decreased vision.

Should any of these occur, contact lenses should immediately be removed. If symptoms persist or worsen after contact lenses have been removed, patients should immediately report to an ophthalmic professional. Patients should also be warned of potential risk factors for corneal infection (e.g. smoking).

The contact lens practitioner must be able to identify an early or potential corneal infection. Any acutely inflamed and painful eye in a patient wearing a contact lens must be considered a medical emergency and the patient should be examined as soon as possible. The observation of an epithelial defect with associated infiltrate, pain and perhaps discharge should immediately suggest infectious keratitis. All contact lens wear should be discontinued (both eyes, to minimize risk of the infection becoming bilateral), and the patient managed appropriately.

Treatment

For many years, academic corneal specialists taught that initial management of suspected microbial corneal infection includes corneal scrapings for stains and cultures to (1) identify the offending pathogen, and (2) determine its sensitivities to various antibiotics. Immediate microscopic examination of stained slides often assists in early identification. Treatment with antibiotics before culturing is known to decrease the potential information gathered from such laboratory investigations and thus complicate later care, should the corneal infection worsen despite initial treatment. Culture media should include blood and chocolate agar, as well as Sabouraud's and thioglycolate media. Jones advocates initiation of antibiotic treatment of bacterial keratitis based on the immediate Gram's stain results, while Baum suggests a broad-spectrum 'shotgun' approach while awaiting results of laboratory investigations to assist in refinement of the treatment if needed (Jones and Baum, 1979).

Although most academic corneal specialists still agree that cultures should be obtained before initiating medical therapy, some have questioned the need for laboratory investigations (smears, stains, cultures and antibiotic sensitivity testing) before initiating treatment, especially for small infiltrates or even 'less severe ulcers' off the visual axis (McDonnell *et al.*, 1992; McLeod *et al.*, 1996a,b; Rodman *et al.*, 1997) (Figure 2.6).

All contact lens-associated corneal infection should be considered as due to *P. aeruginosa* until proven otherwise because of the prevalence of this bacterium in positive cultures and because of its potential catastrophic course without appropriate intervention. The use of topical steroids and patching should therefore not be considered for initial management for any contact lens-associated epithelial defect (Dohlman *et al.*, 1973; Clemons *et al.*, 1987). Both appear to worsen the course of any infectious process, especially those of *Pseudomonas* spp., herpes and fungi.

Presumed bacterial corneal infections have been treated with broad-spectrum antibiotics with both good Gram-negative and Gram-positive bacterial coverage, combinations of cephalosporins (semisynthetic agents chemically related to the penicillins) and aminoglycosides (such as gentamicin and tobramycin) in fortified form (Figure 2.7). Specially prepared ophthalmic formulations of vancomycin are used to treat resistant Gram-positive bacterial infections. New ophthalmic commercial-strength fluoroquinolone preparations have shown excellent *in vitro* activity against many common corneal pathogens, and have also proven

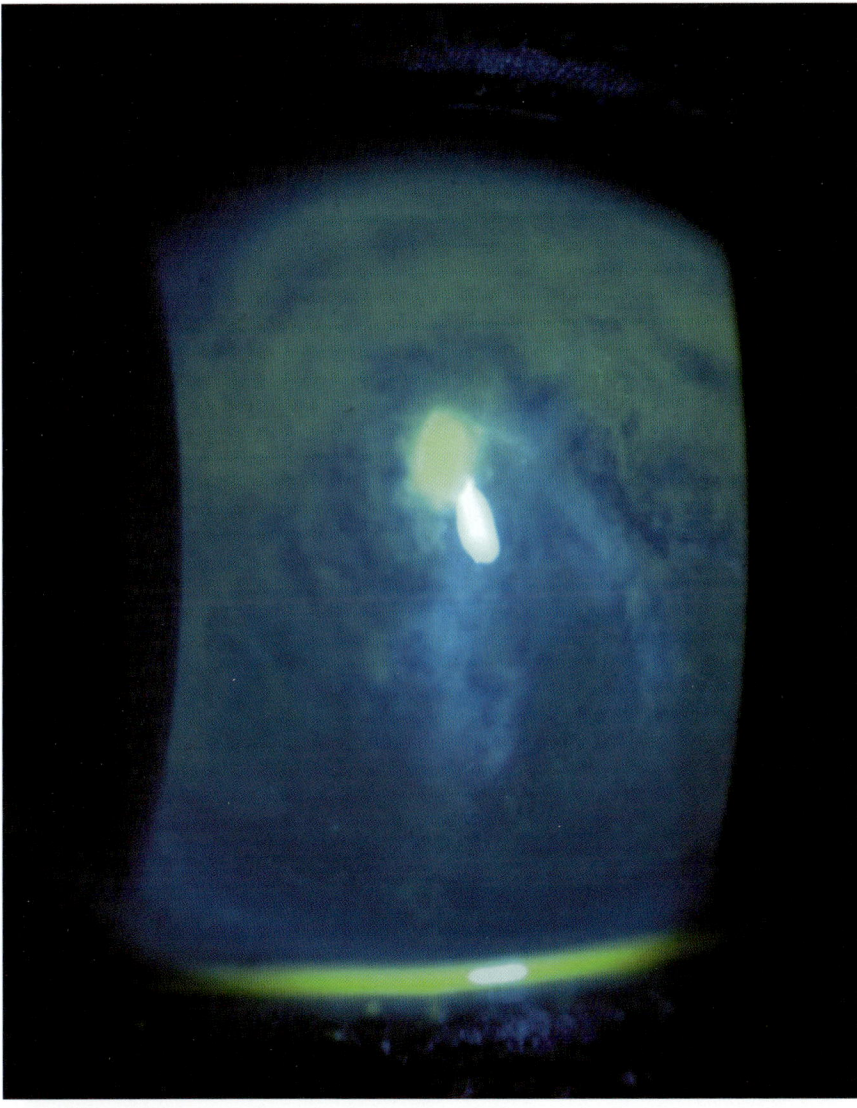

Figure 2.6 Epithelial abrasion with mild infiltration seen in the eye of a keratoconic patient who wore piggyback contact lens systems. This lesion was effectively treated with topical antibiotics

effective in treating keratitis as monotherapy with few adverse reactions (Steinert, 1991; Leibowitz, 1991; O'Brien *et al.*, 1995; Ofloxacin Study Group, 1997). Unfortunately, however, resistance is emerging, leading to treatment failures (Figure 2.8) (Blanton *et al.*, 1996; Knauf *et al.*, 1996).

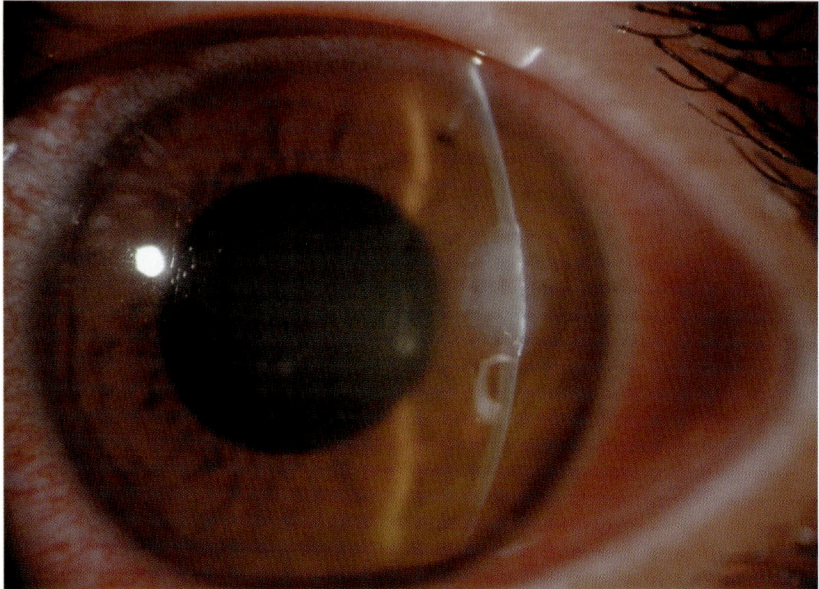

Figure 2.7 Eye with presumed bacterial corneal infections secondary to contact lens wear. This corneal ulcer was culture negative and healed with aggressive topical antibiotic treatment

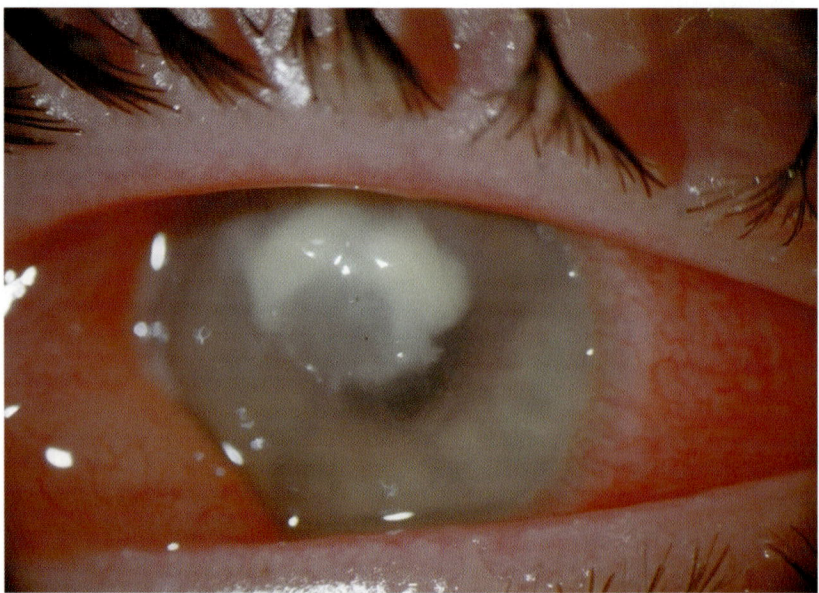

Figure 2.8 This advanced corneal ulcer displays the 'soupy' appearance typical of Gram-negative bacterial keratitis; the lesion was culture positive for *Pseudomonas aeruginosa*

Clinicians may need to reconsider the use of dual therapy in the near future.

The clinician should always consider the possibility of *Acanthamoeba* spp. infections in any contact lens related keratitis, especially chronic disease with initially negative culture results and failure of antibiotic therapy. Clinician suspicion should be increased when (1) the patient reports extreme ocular pain and/or a history of exposure of the contact lenses to non-sterile water, and (2) slit lamp examination reveals the presence of an unusual epitheliopathy (reminiscent of herpetic epithelial disease) and/or a peripheral corneal radial neuropathy.

Special culture techniques are available for *Acanthamoeba* infections, but tissue biopsy is often necessary. Combinations of the following four types of pharmacological agents have been used successfully for medical treatment of *Acanthamoeba* keratitis (Berger *et al.*, 1990; D'Aversa *et al.*, 1995):

1. antibiotic/aminoglycosides – paromomycin, neomycin;
2. antifungal agents – clotrimazole, ketoconazole, itraconazole, miconazole, fluconazole;
3. antiparasitic/aromatic diamidine – propamidine isethionate, hydroxystilbamidine, hexamidine di-isethionate;
4. biocide/cationic antiseptic – polyhexamethylene biguanide, chlorhexidine gluconate, povidone-iodine.

Misdiagnosis and medical failures are common (Groden and Brinser, 1986).

Fungal corneal infections are extremely rare during cosmetic contact lens wear. Most cases reported in the literature involved the use of bandage contact lenses, and/or chronic treatment with topical steroids, in patients suffering from some concurrent ocular disease (e.g. neurotrophic epithelial defects, diabetes, traumatic cases) (Kent *et al.*, 1990). Antifungal pharmaceutical agents are available, but medical treatment is often quite difficult and prone to failure. Clinicians should be aware that atypical mycobacterial and *Acanthamoeba* infections often mimic fungal corneal ulcers and vice versa.

Concomitant viral corneal infections, of which adenovirus and herpes simplex virus are of principal concern, can occur during contact lens wear. No aetiological association has been uncovered for such viral infections, but contact lens wear should usually be discontinued during viral infections unless the contact lens is being used in a treatment protocol. Adenovirus infection is usually successfully managed by supportive therapy such as tear supplements and topical decongestants, or steroid therapy, as the clinical condition indicates. It is often prudent to discard (or disinfect) contact lenses that have been worn during the period of viral infection and dispense new contact lenses, if possible, once the infection has resolved. Effective antiviral agents are available for treatment of herpetic eye disease. The clinician who observes an apparent herpetic keratitis in association with use of contact lenses must always consider the possibility of *Acanthamoeba* as an alternative infectious agent.

Initial treatment is often modified by the clinical course and by the identification and sensitivity of causative microbes isolated by culture and stain results. Some patients, especially those with severe infections and those who are suspected of being potentially non-compliant, should be hospitalized. Persistent and refractory corneal infections may require subconjunctival depot antibiotics (where the medicine slowly leaks back out through the needle tract to bathe the anterior segment of the eye), use of collagen shields presoaked in antibiotics, iontophoresis, systemic treatment, or tectonic corneal transplantation to remove the large reservoir of microbial colonization (and thereby improve the effectiveness of medical management). The positioning of a conjunctival flap may be indicated to encourage healing of a sterilized but persistent epithelial defect. Referral to a specialist with cornea-external eye disease training to manage more severe inflammatory/infectious ocular disease is usually prudent.

Bacteria are eliminated from corneal tissue by both pharmacological and host defence mechanisms. A general optimal duration of antibiotic therapy has not been established, and may indeed vary with different bacterial strains and individual human immunological responses. All viable bacteria are usually killed with one week of topical therapy; *S. epidermidis* infections can even heal in five days. It should be emphasized, however, that corneal ulcers caused by *Pseudomonas* can take more than three weeks of treatment to heal (D'Aversa *et al.*, 1995). Bacterial components and undigested bacteria may remain at the infection site and inside neutrophils to stimulate continued host responses long after all viable microorganisms have been killed.

Patients who respond well to antimicrobial treatment are usually considered healed when the epithelial defect closes and other signs and symptoms decline. The damaged anterior limiting lamina (Bowman's membrane) is replaced by a fibrovascular pannus and necrotic tissue is sloughed away. Complete re-epithelialization can be followed by formation of an opaque and often vascularized scar. With improvements in the contact lens material and design, the use of better care systems, the adoption of more appropriate patterns of use, and the introduction of strategies to reduce the risk of recurrence, refitting of contact lenses may be reconsidered, and may even be indicated for visual rehabilitation, perhaps six weeks after the eye has become stable and quiet.

Summary

Corneal infection is a rare but potentially serious complication of contact lens wear. Certainly, contact lens wear – especially extended wear – has become an important known risk factor in corneal infection. Bacteria (particularly *Pseudomonas* spp. and *Staphylococcus* spp.) are the most common microbes isolated from corneal infections after cosmetic contact lens wear, followed by *Acanthamoeba* spp. (protozoa) and rarely fungi. Therapeutic (bandage) contact lens use is also potentially hazardous, and the clinician that follows such patients must be particularly alert for fungal or Gram-positive infections. Viral corneal infections also occur concomitant with contact lens wear but there does not appear to be any aetiological linkage. Clinically, observation of a corneal epithelial defect and associated infiltrate, in a setting of pain and discharge and with a history of contact lens wear, must be presumed to be a microbial corneal infection until proven otherwise. Such an event must be treated as a medical emergency. Management consists initially of prevention, but in the event that signs or symptoms appear, an immediate response, a rapid diagnosis, and the employment of appropriate therapeutic action is essential.

References

Adams, C. P., Cohen, E. J., Laibson, P. R. *et al.* (1983) Corneal ulcers in patients with cosmetic extended-wear contact lenses. *Am. J. Ophthalmol.*, **96**, 705–709.

Alvord, L., Court, J., Davis, T. *et al.* (1998) Oxygen permeability of a new type of high Dk soft contact lens material. *Optom. Vis. Sci.*, **75**, 30–36.

Bates, A. K., Morris, R. J., Stapleton, F. *et al.* (1989) 'Sterile' corneal infiltrates in contact lens wearers. *Eye*, **3**, 803–810.

Baum, J. L. and Panjwani, N. (1988) Adherence of *Pseudomonas* to soft contact lenses and cornea: mechanisms and prophylaxis. In *The Cornea: Transactions of the World Congress on the Cornea III* (H. Cavanagh, ed.) pp. 301–307, Raven Press.

Belmont, J. B., Ostler, H. B., Dawson, C. R. *et al.* (1982) Non-infectious ring-shaped keratitis associated with Pseudomonas aeruginosa. *Am. J. Ophthalmol.*, **93**, 338–341.

Berger, S. T., Mondino, B. J., Hoft, R. H. *et al.* (1990) Successful management of acanthamoeba keratitis. *Am. J. Ophthalmol.*, **110**, 395–403.

Bergmanson, J. P., Ruben, C. M. and Chu, L. W. (1985) Epithelial morphological response to soft hydrogel contact lenses. *Br. J. Ophthalmol.*, **69**, 373–379.

Binder, P. S. and Woodward, C. (1980) Extended-wear Hydrocurve and Sauflon contact lenses. *Am. J. Ophthalmol.*, **90**, 309–316.

Blanton, C. L., Rapuano, C. J., Cohen, E. J. *et al.* (1996) Initial treatment of microbial keratitis. *Contact Lens Assoc. Ophthalmol. J.*, **22**, 136–140.

Brown, S. I., Bloomfield, S., Pearce, D. B. and Tragakis, M. (1974) Infections with the therapeutic soft lens. *Arch. Ophthalmol.*, **91**, 275–277.

Campbell, R. C. and Caroline, P. J. (1990) Inefficacy of soft contact lens disinfection techniques in the home environment. *Contact Lens Forum*, **15**, 17–26.

Chalupa, E., Swarbrick, H. A., Holden, B. A. and Sjöstrand, J. (1987) Severe corneal infections associated with contact lens wear. *Ophthalmology*, **94**, 17–31.

Chan, W. K. and Weissman, B. A. (1996) Corneal pannus associated with contact lens wear. *Am. J. Ophthalmol.*, **121**, 540–546.

Cheung, K. H., Laung, S. L., Hoekman, H. W. *et al.* (1999) Incidence of contact lens associated microbial keratitis and its related morbidity. *Lancet*, **354**, 181–185.

Chun, M. W. and Weissman, B. A. (1987) Compliance in contact lens care. *Am. J. Optom. Physiol. Opt.*, **64**, 274–276.

Chynn, E. W., Talamo, J. H. and Seligman, M. S. (1997) Acanthamoeba keratitis: is water exposure a true risk factor? *Contact Lens Assoc. Ophthalmol. J.*, **23**, 55–56.

Claydon, B. E. and Efron, N. (1994) Non-compliance in contact lens wear. *Ophthal. Physiol. Opt.*, **14**, 356–364.

Claydon, B. E., Efron, N. and Woods, C. A. (1997) A prospective study of the effect of education on non-compliant behaviour in contact lens wear. *Ophthal. Physiol. Opt.*, **17**, 137–146.

Clemons, C. S., Cohen, E. J., Arentsen, J. J. *et al.* (1987) Pseudomonas ulcers following patching of corneal abrasions associated with contact lens wear. *Contact Lens Assoc. Ophthalmol. J.*, **13**, 161–164.

Collins, M. J. and Carney, L. G. (1986) Patient compliance and its influence on contact lens wearing problems. *Am. J. Optom. Physiol. Opt.*, **63**, 952–956.

Cooper, R. L. and Constable, I. J. (1977) Infective keratitis in soft contact lens wearers. *Br. J. Ophthalmol.*, **61**, 250–254.

Cutter, G. R., Chalmers, R. L. and Roseman, M. (1996) The clinical presentation, prevalence, and risk factors of focal corneal infiltrates in soft contact lens wearers. *Contact Lens Assoc. Ophthalmol. J.*, **22**, 30–37.

D'Aversa, G., Stern, G. A. and Driebe, W. T. (1995) Diagnosis and successful treatment of acanthamoeba keratitis. *Arch. Ophthalmol.*, **113**, 1120–1123.

Dixon, J. M., Young, C. A., Baldone, J. A. *et al.* (1966) Complications associated with the wearing of contact lenses. *J. Am. Med. Assoc.*, **195**, 901–903.

Dohlman, C. H., Boruchoff, A. and Mobilia, E. F. (1973) Complications in use of soft contact lenses in corneal disease. *Arch. Ophthalmol.*, **90**, 367–371.

Donshik, P. C., Suchecki, J. K. and Ehlers, W. H. (1995) Peripheral corneal infiltrates associated with contact lens wear. *Trans. Am. Ophthalmol. Soc.*, **93**, 49–60.

Donzis, P. B. (1998) Corneal ulcers from contact lenses during travel to remote areas (letter). *N. Engl. J. Med.*, **338**, 1629–1630.

Donzis, P. B., Mondino, B. J., Weissman, B. A. and Bruckner, D.A. (1987) Microbial contamination of contact lens care systems. *Am. J. Ophthalmol.*, **104**, 325–333.

Donzis, P. B., Mondino, B. J. and Weissman, B. A. (1988) Bacillus keratitis associated with contaminated contact lens care systems. *Am. J. Ophthalmol.*, **105**, 195–197.

Efron, N. (1999) *Contact Lens Complications*. Butterworth-Heinemann/Optician.

Efron, N. and Ang, J. H. B. (1990) Corneal hypoxia and hypercapnia during contact lens wear. *Optom. Vis. Sci.*, **67**, 512–521.

Efron, N. and Carney, L. G. (1979) Oxygen levels beneath the closed eyelid. *Invest. Ophthalmol. Vis. Sci.*, **18**, 93–95.

Eichenbaum, J. W., Feldstein, M. and Podos, S. M. (1982) Extended-wear aphakic soft contact lenses and corneal ulcers. *Br. J. Ophthalmol.*, **66**, 663–666.

Fleiszig, S. M., Lee, E. J., Wu, C. *et al.* (1998) Cytotoxic strains of *Pseudomonas aeruginosa* can damage the intact corneal surface in vitro. *Contact Lens Assoc. Ophthalmol. J.*, **24**, 41–47.

Freedman, H. and Sugar, J. (1976) Pseudomonas keratitis following cosmetic soft contact lens wear. *Contact Lens J.*, **10**, 21–25.

Fujikawa, L. S., Salahuddin, S. Z., Ablashi, D. *et al.* (1986) HTLV-III in the tears of AIDS patients. *Ophthalmology*, **93**, 1479–1481.

Garwood, P. C. (1991) Complications with daily wear disposable contact lenses. *Contact Lens J.*, **19**, 137–141.

Gasparrini, E. (1893) Il diplocco di Frankel in patologia oculare: studio sperimentale e clinico. *Ann. Ottol.*, **22**, 131–134.

Gordon, A. and Kracher, G. P. (1985) Corneal infiltrates and extended-wear contact lenses. *J. Am Optom. Assoc.*, **56**, 198–201.

Grant, T., Chong, M. S., Vajdic, C. *et al.* (1998) Contact lens induced peripheral ulcers during hydrogel contact lens wear. *Contact Lens Assoc. Ophthalmol. J.*, **24**, 145–50.

Groden, L. R. and Brinser, J. H. (1986) Outpatient treatment of microbial corneal ulcers. *Arch. Ophthalmol*, **104**, 84–86.

Groden, L. R., Pascucci, S. E., Brinser, J. H. (1987) *Haemophilus aphrophilus* as a cause of crystalline keratopathy. *Am. J. Ophthalmol.*, **104**, 89–90.

Hartstein, J. (1982) *Extended Wear Contact Lenses for Aphakia and Myopia*. C. V. Mosby.

Herman, J. (1987) Clinical management of GPC. *Contact Lens Spectrum*, **2**, 24–33.

Hirji, N. K. and Larke, J. R. (1979) Corneal thickness in extended wear of soft contact lenses. *Br. J. Ophthalmol.*, **63**, 274–276.

Holden, B. A. and Mertz, G. W. (1984) Critical oxygen levels to avoid corneal oedema for daily and extended wear contact lenses. *Invest. Ophthalmol. Vis. Sci.*, **25**, 1161–1167.

Holden, B. A., Sweeney, D. F. and Sanderson, G. (1984) The minimum precorneal oxygen tension to avoid corneal oedema. *Invest. Ophthalmol. Vis. Sci.*, **25**, 476–480.

Holden, B. A., Reddy, M. K., Sankaridurg, P. R. *et al.* (1999) Contact lens induced peripheral ulcers with extended wear of disposable hydrogel lenses; histopathologic observations on the nature and type of corneal infiltrate. *Cornea*, **18**, 538–543.

Hyndiuk, R. A. (1981) Experimental Pseudomonas keratitis. *Trans. Am. Ophthalmol. Soc.*, **79**, 540–624.

Imayasu, M., Petroll, W. M., Jester, J. V. *et al.* (1994) The relation between contact lens oxygen transmissibility and binding of *Pseudomonas aeruginosa* to the cornea after overnight wear. *Ophthalmology*, **101**, 371–388.

Isenberg, S. J. and Green, B. F. (1985) Changes in conjunctival oxygen tension and temperature with advancing age. *Crit. Care Med.*, **13**, 683–685.

Jones, D. B. (1978) Pathogenesis of bacterial and fungal keratitis. *Trans. Ophthalmol. Soc. UK*, **98**, 367–371.

Jones, D. B. (1981) Decision-making in the management of microbial keratitis. *Ophthalmology*, **88**, 814–820.

Jones, D. B. and Baum, J. L. (1979) Initial therapy of suspected microbial corneal ulcers. I. Broad antibiotic therapy based on prevalence of organisms. *Surv. Ophthalmol.*, **24**, 97–105.

Kent, H. D., Cohen, E. J., Laibson, P. R. and Arentsen, J. J. (1990) Microbial keratitis and corneal ulceration associated with therapeutic soft contact lenses. *Contact Lens Assoc. Ophthalmol. J.*, **16**, 49–52.

Kenyon, E., Polse, K. A. and Seger, R. G. (1986) Influence of wearing schedule on extended-wear complications. *Ophthalmology*, **93**, 231–236.

Knauf, H. P., Silvany, R., Southern, P. M. Jr *et al.* (1996) Susceptibility of corneal and conjunctival pathogens to ciprofloxacin. *Cornea*, **15**, 66–71.

Koenig, S. B., Solomon, J. M., Hyndiuk, R. A. *et al.* (1987) Acanthamoeba keratitis associated with gas-permeable contact lens wear. *Am. J. Ophthalmol.*, **103**, 832.

Krachmer, J. H. and Purcell, J. J. Jr (1978) Bacterial corneal ulcers in cosmetic soft contact lens wearers. *Arch. Ophthalmol.*, **96**, 57–61.

Larke, J. R. and Hirji, N. K. (1979) Some clinically observed phenomena in extended contact lens wear. *Br. J. Ophthalmol.*, **63**, 475–477.

Larke, J. R., Parrish, S. T. and Wigham, C. G. (1981) Apparent human corneal oxygen uptake rate. *Am. J. Optom. Physiol. Opt.*, **58**, 803–805.

Leibowitz, H. M. (1991) Clinical evaluation of ciprofloxacin 0.3% ophthalmic solution for treatment of bacterial keratitis. *Am. J. Ophthalmol.*, **112**, 34S–47S.

Locatcher-Khorazo, D., Seegal, B. C. and Gutierrez, E. H. (1972a) Bacterial infections of the eye. In *Microbiology of the Eye* (D. Locatcher-Khorazo and B. C. Seegal, eds), pp. 63–72, C. V. Mosby.

Locatcher-Khorazo, D., Seegal, B. C. and Gutierrez, E. H. (1972b) The bacterial flora of the healthy eye. In *Microbiology of the Eye* (D. Locatcher-Khorazo and B. C. Seegal, eds), pp. 13–23, C. V. Mosby.

MacRae, S., Herman, C., Stulting, R. D. *et al.* (1991) Corneal ulcer and adverse reaction rates in premarket contact lens studies. *Am. J. Ophthalmol.*, **111**, 457–465.

Mandell, R. B. and Farrell, R. (1980) Corneal swelling at low atmospheric oxygen pressures. *Invest. Ophthalmol. Vis. Sci.*, **19**, 697–702.

McDonnell, P. J., Nobe, J., Gauderman, W. J. *et al.* (1992) Community care of corneal ulcers. *Am. J. Ophthalmol.*, **114**, 531–538.

McLeod, S. D., DeBacker, C. M. and Viana, M. A. (1996a) Differential care of corneal ulcers in the community based on apparent severity. *Ophthalmology*, **103**, 479–484.

McLeod, S. D., Kolahdouz-Isfahani, A., Rostamian, K., *et al.* (1996b) The role of smears, cultures and antibiotic sensitivity testing in the management of suspected infectious keratitis. *Ophthalmology*, **103**, 23–28.

Meisler, D. M., Langston, R. H., Naab, T. J. *et al.* (1984) Infectious crystalline keratopathy. *Am. J. Ophthalmol.*, **97**, 337–343.

Mondino, B. J. and Dethlefs, B. (1984) Occurrence of phlyctenules after immunization with ribitol teichoic acid of *Staphylococcus aureus*. *Arch. Ophthalmol.*, **102**, 461–463.

Mondino, B. J and Groden, L. R. (1980) Conjunctival hyperemia and corneal infiltrates with chemically disinfected soft contact lenses. *Arch. Ophthalmol.*, **98**, 1767–1770.

Mondino, B. J., Weissman, B. A., Farb, M. D. and Pettit, T. H. (1986) Corneal ulcers associated with daily-wear and extended-wear contact lenses. *Am. J. Ophthalmol.*, **102**, 58–65.

Moore, M. B., McCulley, J. P., Luckenbach, M. *et al.* (1985) Acanthamoeba keratitis associated with soft contact lenses. *Am. J. Ophthalmol.*, **100**, 396–403.

Moore, M. B., McCulley, J. P., Newton, C. *et al.* (1987) Acanthamoeba keratitis. A growing problem in soft and hard contact lens wearers. *Ophthalmology*, **94**, 1654–1661.

Naginton, J., Watson, P. G., Playfair, T. J. *et al.* (1974) Amoebic infection of the eye. *Lancet*, **ii** (7896), 1537–1540.

Nanda, M., Pflugfelder, S. C. and Holland, S. (1991) Fulminant pseudomonal keratitis and scleritis in human immunodeficiency virus-infected patients. *Arch. Ophthalmol.*, **109**, 503–505.

O'Brien, T. P., Maguire, M. G., Fink, N. E. *et al.* (1995) Efficacy of ofloxacin vs cefazolin and tobramycin in the therapy for bacterial keratitis. Report from the Bacterial Keratitis Study Research Group. *Arch. Ophthalmol.*, **113**, 1257–1265.

O'Donnell, C., Efron, N. and Boulton, A. J. M. (2001) A prospective study of contact lens wear in diabetes mellitus. *Ophthal. Physiol. Opt.*, **21**, 127–138.

Ofloxacin Study Group (1997) Ofloxacin monotherapy for the primary treatment of microbial keratitis: a double-masked, randomized, controlled trial with conventional therapy. *Ophthalmology*, **104**, 1902–1909.

Ogawa, G. S. H. and Hyndiuk, R. K. (1994) Bacterial keratitis and conjunctivitis; clinical disease. In *The Cornea*, 3rd edn (G. Smolin and R. A. Thoft, eds), pp. 125–168, Little Brown.

O'Leary, D. J. and Millodot, M. (1981) Abnormal epithelial fragility in diabetes and contact lens wear. *Acta Ophthalmol.*, **59**, 827–833.

Ormerod, L. D. and Smith, R. E. (1986) Contact lens-associated microbial keratitis. *Arch. Ophthalmol.*, **104**, 79–83.

Penley, C. A., Llabrés, C., Wilson, L. A. and Ahearn, D. G. (1985) Efficacy of hydrogen peroxide disinfection systems for soft contact lenses contaminated with fungi. *Contact Lens Assoc. Ophthalmol. J.*, **11**, 65–68.

Pitts, R. E. and Krachmer, J. H. (1979) Evaluation of soft contact lens disinfection in the home environment. *Arch. Ophthalmol.*, **97**, 470–472.

Poggio, E. C., Glynn, R. J., Schein, O. D. *et al.* (1989) The incidence of ulcerative keratitis among users of daily-wear and extended-wear soft contact lenses. *N. Engl. J. Med.*, **321**, 779–783.

Polse, K. A. and Mandell, R. B. (1970) Critical oxygen tension at the corneal surface. *Arch. Ophthalmol.*, **84**, 505–508.

Ramphal, R., McNiece, M. T. and Polack, F. M. (1981) Adherence of *Pseudomonas aeruginosa* to the injured cornea: a step in the pathogenesis of corneal infections. *Ann. Ophthalmol.*, **13**, 421–425.

Reiss, G. R., Campbell, R. J. and Bourne, W. M. (1986) Infectious crystalline keratopathy. *Surv. Ophthalmol.*, **31**, 69–72.

Rodman, R. C., Spisak, S., Sugar, A. *et al.* (1997) The utility of culturing corneal ulcers in a tertiary referral center versus a general ophthalmology clinic. *Ophthalmology*, **104**, 1897–1901.

Rozenman, Y., Donnenfeld, E. D., Cohen, E. J. *et al.* (1989) Contact lens related deep stromal neovascularization. *Am. J. Ophthalmol.*, **107**, 27–32.

Ruben, M. (1976) Acute eye disease secondary to contact-lens wear. *Lancet*, **1** (7951), 138–140.

Salz, J. J. and Schlanger, J. L. (1983) Complications of aphakic extended wear lenses encountered during a seven-year period in 100 eyes. *Contact Lens Assoc. Ophthalmol. J.*, **9**, 241–244.

Sankaridurg, P. R., Sharma, S., Willcox, M. *et al.* (1999a) Colonization of hydrogel lenses with *Streptococcus pneumoniae*: risk of development of corneal infiltrates. *Cornea*, **18**, 289–295.

Sankaridurg, P. R., Sweeney, D. F., Sharma, S. *et al.* (1999b) Adverse events with extended wear of disposable hydrogels: results for the first 13 months of lens wear. *Ophthalmology*, **106**, 1671–1680.

Schein, O. D., Glynn, R. J., Poggio, E. C. *et al.* (1989a) The relative risk of ulcerative keratitis among users of daily-wear and extended-wear soft contact lenses. A case control study. Microbial Keratitis Study Group. *N. Engl. J. Med.*, **321**, 773–778.

Schein, O. D., Ormerod, L. D., Barraquer, E. *et al.* (1989b) Microbiology of contact lens-related keratitis. *Cornea*, **8**, 281–285.

Shah, S. S., Yeung, K. K. and Weissman, B. A. (1998) Contact lens deep stromal vascularization. *Int. Contact Lens Clin.*, **25**, 128–136.

Spoor, T. C., Hartel, W. C., Wynn, P. and Spoor, D. K. (1984) Complications of continuous-wear soft contact lenses in a nonreferral population. *Arch. Ophthalmol.*, **102**, 1312–1313.

Stark, W. J. and Martin, N. F. (1981) Extended-wear contact lenses for myopic correction. *Arch. Ophthalmol.*, **99**, 1963–1966.

Stark, W. J., Kracher, G. P., Cowen, C. L. *et al.* (1979) Extended-wear contact lenses and intraocular lenses for aphakic correction. *Am. J. Ophthalmol.*, **88**, 535–542.

Stehr-Green, J. K, Bailey, T. M. and Visvesvara, G. S. (1988) The epidemiology of Acanthamoeba keratitis in the United States. *Am. J. Ophthalmol.*, **107**, 331–336.

Stein, R. M., Clinch, T. E., Cohen, E. J. *et al.* (1988) Infected vs sterile corneal infiltrates in contact lens wearers. *Am. J. Ophthalmol.*, **105**, 632–636.

Steinert, R. F. (1991) Current therapy for bacterial keratitis and bacterial conjunctivitis. *Am. J. Ophthalmol.*, **112**, 10S–14S.

Stern, G. A., Weitzenkorn, D. and Valenti, J. (1982) Adherence of *Pseudomonas aeruginosa* to the mouse cornea. Epithelial v stromal adherence. *Arch. Ophthalmol.*, **100**, 1956–1958.

Stern, G. A., Lubniewski, A. and Allen, C. (1985) The interaction between *Pseudomonas aeruginosa* and the corneal epithelium. An electron microscopic study. *Arch. Ophthalmol.*, **103**, 1221–1225.

Weissman, B. A., Mondino, B. J., Pettit, T. H. and Hofbauer, J. D. (1984) Corneal ulcers associated with extended-wear soft contact lenses. *Am. J. Ophthalmol.*, **97**, 476–481.

Weissman, B. A., Donzis, P. B. and Hoft, R. H. (1987a) Keratitis and contact lens wear: a review. *J. Am. Optom. Assoc.*, **58**, 799–803.

Weissman, B. A., Remba, M. J. and Fugedy, E. (1987b) Results of the extended wear contact lens survey of the Contact Lens Section of the American Optometric Association. *J. Am. Optom. Assoc.*, **58**, 166–171.

Weissman, B. A., Chun, M. W. and Barnhart, L. A. (1994) Corneal abrasion associated with correction of keratoconus – a retrospective study. *Optom. Vis. Sci.*, **71**, 677–681.

Wilcox, M. D., Power, K. N., Stapleton, F. *et al..* (1997) Potential sources of bacteria that are isolated from contact lenses during wear. *Optom. Vis. Sci.,* **74,** 1030–1038.

Wilhelmus, K. R. (1987) Review of clinical experience with microbial keratitis associated with contact lenses. *Contact Lens Assoc. Ophthalmol. J.,* **13,** 211–241.

Wilhelmus, K.R. (1996) Bacterial keratitis. In *Ocular Infection and Immunity* (J. S. Pepose, G. H. Holland and K. R. Wilhemus, eds), pp. 970–1031, Mosby-Yearbook.

Wilson, L. A. and Ahearn, D. G. (1986) Association of fungi with extended-wear soft contact lenses. *Am. J. Ophthalmol.,* **101,** 434–436.

Wilson, L. A., Schlitzer, R. L. and Ahearn, D. G. (1981) Pseudomonas corneal ulcers associated with soft contact-lens wear. *Am. J. Ophthalmol.,* **92,** 546–554.

Zantos, S. D. and Holden, B. A. (1978) Ocular changes associated with continuous wear of contact lenses. *Aust. J. Optom.,* **61,** 418–426.

3 Confocal microscopy

Nathan Efron, Jo Hollingsworth, Hui Hiang Koh,
Carole Maldonado-Codina, Philip B. Morgan, Haliza A. Mutalib,
Clare O'Donnell, Laura Oliveira-Soto, Anupa Patel,
Inma Perez-Gomez and Andrew B. Tullo

Introduction

Contact lens practitioners rely on the optical slit lamp biomicroscope in the critical task of examining the anterior ocular structures before, during and after contact lens wear. This instrument is extremely flexible in that it offers a stereoscopic view over a range of magnifications. The cornea can be illuminated with a slit of light that can be tilted and rotated, varied in terms of brightness, width and height, and interposed with coloured and polarizing filters. The full capabilities of the slit lamp for examining contact lens-induced corneal abnormalities have been described in Chapters 1 and 2.

A critical limitation of the slit lamp is that the highest practicable magnification possible is around 40×, with a lateral resolution of 30 µm. In certain circumstances, this places a considerable constraint upon clinical decision-making. For example, in Chapter 2, Weissman and Mondino highlight the difficulty in effecting a differential diagnosis when confronted with a sore, red eye and hazy cornea. What is required is a technique that enables examination of such a condition at very high magnification, so that tissue structures can be viewed at a cellular level and extraneous matter such as infectious agents can be identified. Of course, extremely high magnification is available with scanning and transmission electron microscopes, but these techniques only allow examination of excised tissue. The application of electron microscopy in studies of contact lens-induced corneal pathology is discussed by Bergmanson in Chapter 4.

The relatively new technique of confocal microscopy offers clinicians the opportunity to examine the living human cornea at a magnification of around 680× (Figure 3.1). In this chapter, the optical principle of confocal microscopy will be described, and the development of this instrument will be recounted up to present time, when confocal microscopy is becoming a viable clinical technique. The design and construction of current instruments will be outlined. A qualitative and

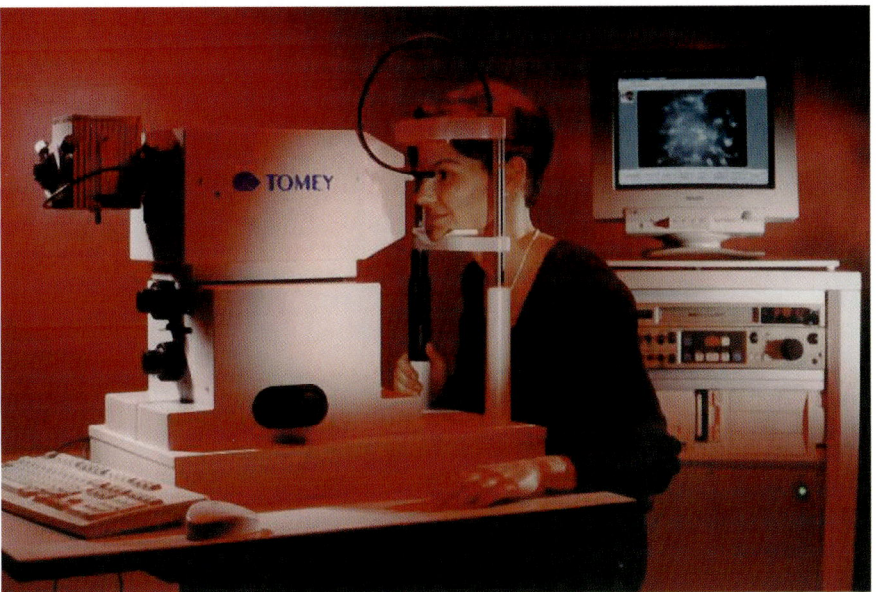

Figure 3.1 The Tomey ConfoScan P4 *in vivo* slit-scanning real-time confocal microscope (Courtesy of Maldonado-Codina and O'Donnell, 1999)

quantitative analysis of images obtained from normal human corneas using this technique will be presented, along with the results of preliminary research detailing the effects of contact lens wear on the cornea.

Optical principles

In broad terms, the optical principle of the confocal microscope is that field of view is sacrificed for resolution. In the slit lamp, a broad beam of light is used to view a large section of cornea at relatively low magnification. This arrangement offers a large field of view, but resolution is limited. With the confocal microscope, the opposite situation occurs. A tiny spot of light is projected into the cornea, and this illuminated spot of corneal tissue is viewed simultaneously. This results in very high resolution but virtually no field of view. Of course, an instrument offering a negligible field of view would not be much use; the confocal microscope solves this problem by instantaneously illuminating a small region of the cornea with thousands of tiny spots of light each second, with each spot of light being synchronously imaged. The spot images are reconstructed to create a usable field of view offering high resolution and magnification.

In the confocal microscope, therefore, a single point in the tissue is both optically illuminated from a point light source and simultaneously imaged by a point detector; i.e. they are in the same focal plane, or 'confocal' (Figure 3.2). Any adjacent features in the tissue outside the

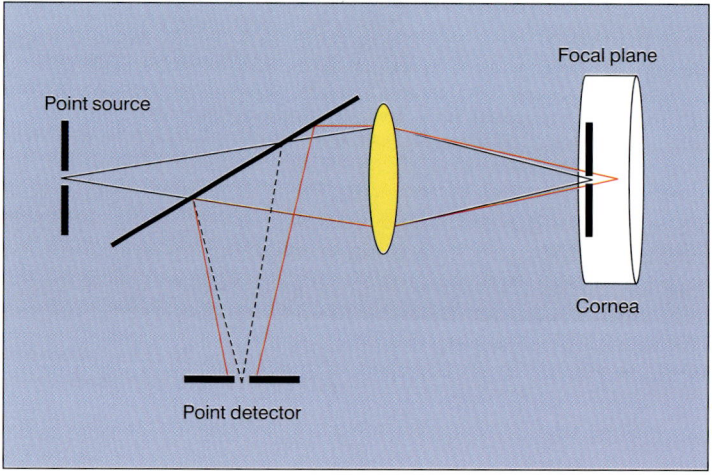

Figure 3.2 Optical principle of the confocal microscope (Courtesy of Maldonado-Codina and O'Donnell, 1999)

plane of interest are attenuated. This results in an image of good contrast with high levels of lateral and axial resolution.

The high axial (or depth) resolution is responsible for the confocal microscope being described as an instrument that is capable of 'optically sectioning' the cornea. That is, as the instrument is focused in and out of the cornea, a section only about 10 μm thick is observed at any one time. This sectioning capability is essential because structures of interest to be viewed in the cornea at a cellular level, such as epithelial cells, stromal keratocytes, corneal nerves and endothelial cells, scatter or reflect light weakly. Optical sectioning allows these structures to be viewed in good contrast against a dark background. It is important to emphasize that the 'sections' being viewed are *en face*, or 'front on', which means that only one layer of corneal tissue is observed in any given image. This is unlike the more common histological form of corneal sectioning whereby the cornea is cut from the front to back and all corneal layers can be observed in a single cross-section of tissue.

Historical development

The concept of the confocal microscope can be traced back to 1957 when Minsky filed a patent for a such an instrument to examine excised neural tissue from the brain (Minsky, 1988). The early designs utilized a spinning Nipkow disc – a device that contained thousands of sets of conjugate pinholes, each 40–60 μm in diameter, arranged in several sets of Archimedes spirals; i.e. each pinhole on one side of the disc has a conjugate pinhole in the other side of the disc. The illumination light passes through a set of about 100 pinholes and is imaged by a microscope objective to form a diffraction-limited spot on the specimen. The reflected light from the specimen passes through the conjugate set of pinholes on the other side of the disc to form the image. The illuminated and reflected light are effectively scanned across the specimen as the disc rotates and a different set of conjugate pinholes in the Archimedes spiral becomes interposed in the optical system. An instrument constructed in this way is known as a tandem scanning confocal microscope (Böhnke and Masters, 1999).

The spinning Nipkow disc principle was employed by Petran *et al.* in 1968 to construct a real-time, direct view confocal microscope for examining excised corneal tissue. The first breakthrough in terms of observing the cornea of a human patient came when Lemp and colleagues (Lemp *et al.*, 1986) arranged to mount a Petran tandem scanning confocal microscope on a platform with adjacent headrest. Although this early instrument allowed visualization of cellular elements of the living human cornea, it was not suited for routine clinical use for a number of reasons. The Nipkow disc allows only 1% of the incident light to be transmitted. Because the cornea is essentially transparent, the individual corneal elements being viewed reflect little light back. Of this reflected light, only 1% is transmitted back through the Nipkow disc to the ocular or detector. As a result of this gross attenuation of light through the system, the illumination source must be extremely bright, typically employing a xenon or mercury arc lamp; such high levels of illumination are very uncomfortable for the subject being observed, and could indeed result in ocular damage during prolonged examinations. Other disadvantages included the need to physically applanate the cornea with the microscope objective, and the requirement for image enhancement by way of frame averaging to reduce the noise and remove scan lines (which means that the instrument is not operating in real time) (Böhnke and Masters, 1999).

The availability of confocal microscopes suitable for clinical use in the mid–1990s can be attributed to the replacement of the Nipkow disc-mediated multiple point light source system with a slit-scanning device

(Masters and Thaer, 1994). Essentially, the image of a slit is scanned over the back focal plane of the microscope objective. The slit width can be varied in order to optimize the balance of optical section thickness and image brightness. A double-sided mirror is used for scanning and descanning and a halogen lamp is used for illuminating the slit. The detector is a video camera that acquires images at video rates. Another key advantage of the slit scanning device is the employment of a non-applanating, high numerical aperture, water immersion microscope objective, which does not touch the cornea. A methylcellulose gel is used to optically couple the tip of the microscope objective to the cornea (Figure 3.3). The high numerical aperture of the objective lens is

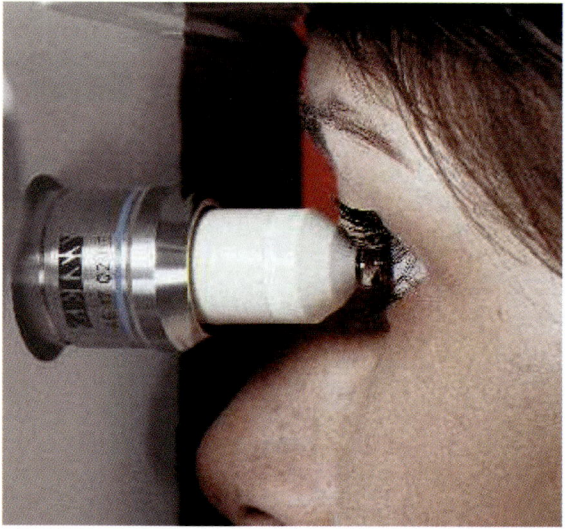

Figure 3.3 Methylcellulose gel coupling the tip of the objective to the cornea (Courtesy of Maldonado-Codina and O'Donnell, 1999)

very efficient in collecting the light from weakly reflecting corneal structures. This allows all of the epithelial layers (superficial, wing and basal cells) to be distinguished, which was not possible with earlier confocal microscopes, which could only image the basal epithelial cell layer.

The main disadvantage of the slit scanning system compared with the pinhole design is that the microscope is only truly confocal in the axis perpendicular to the slit height. The optical ramification of this configuration is that slit-based confocal microscopes provide lower transverse and axial resolution compared with pinhole-based instruments. However, this trade-off – accepting lower resolution in favour of higher light throughput – is acceptable as it has allowed the slit scanning device to be developed into a viable clinical instrument.

More sophisticated applications of the confocal microscope include examination of the cornea under fluorescent light (Hahnel *et al.*, 2000) and the computer-assisted generation of three-dimensional images of corneal elements (Masters and Farmer, 1993; Hahnel *et al.*, 2000), which are reconstructions from serial sections. These applications will not be considered in detail here.

Clinical application

As explained above, the confocal microscope is rapidly evolving from a research laboratory tool into a clinical instrument. It is therefore important that consideration be given to the development of protocols so that the confocal microscope can be used routinely and effectively in a clinical setting. The features and method of use of a confocal microscope designed specifically for this purpose are described below.

Equipment

The instrument used to conduct the research described throughout this chapter is the Tomey ConfoScan P4 in vivo slit-scanning real-time confocal microscope (Erlangen, Germany) (Figure 3.1). A 12 V/100 W halogen lamp provides a steady, even illumination, and filters are enclosed in the lamp housing to screen out excessive ultraviolet and infrared radiation. Twenty-five images are captured each second on a high-sensitivity black-and-white video camera; this capture rate is synchronized to the frequency and phase of the scanning mechanism in order to optimize image quality. The images are viewed in real time on a computer screen and can be stored on video tape for subsequent examination and analysis. The real-time image as seen on the computer screen (or a video replay in real time) is in a rapid state of movement because of the high magnification and small field of view, natural microsaccadic eye movements, and the necessary instrument manipulation (focusing and positioning). It is only via slow motion video replay, or even frame-by-frame advancement, that an overall appreciation of structure of the cornea, and of any abnormalities present, can be gained. High-quality video frames, absent of any blur, can be selected for detailed morphometric analysis.

The cornea is optically coupled to the objective using a viscous gel (Viscotears® Liquid Gel, Ciba Vision) with a refractive index similar to that of the cornea (Figure 3.3). Three different Achroplan® immersion objective lenses are available in magnification/numerical aperture combinations of 20×/0.4, 40×/0.7 and 63×/0.9. An Epiplan® 20×/0.5 non-contact 'dry lens' is also available. We found the Achroplan 40×/0.75NA immersion lens to be most suited for general imaging; this lens gives a field of view of the cornea of 330×240 μm, a depth of visible field of 10 μm, and a lateral resolution of about 1 μm. All of the images displayed in this chapter were obtained using this lens.

The Tomey ConfoScan P4 consists of a number of components. The confocal microscope, halogen lamp, camera, light source and objective lens are enclosed in a common instrument housing, which sits on, and moves independently of, a base-unit that contains X-Y-Z direction controls and an adjustable chin and head rest. The video images are transmitted via a cable to the operation console, which contains a digital video monitor, Super-VHS video recorder and computer.

The instrument can be used in 'confocal microscopy through focusing' (CMTF) mode (also known as 'Z-scan' mode). In this configuration, depth-of-focus information is displayed by way of a profile of scattered light from the cornea (Figure 3.4). The Z-scan is effected by way of a continuously recording photomultiplier. A number of scans from the anterior to the posterior cornea are generated by rapidly oscillating a movable lens within the objective housing backwards and forwards in order to change the focal position within the cornea. The position of the

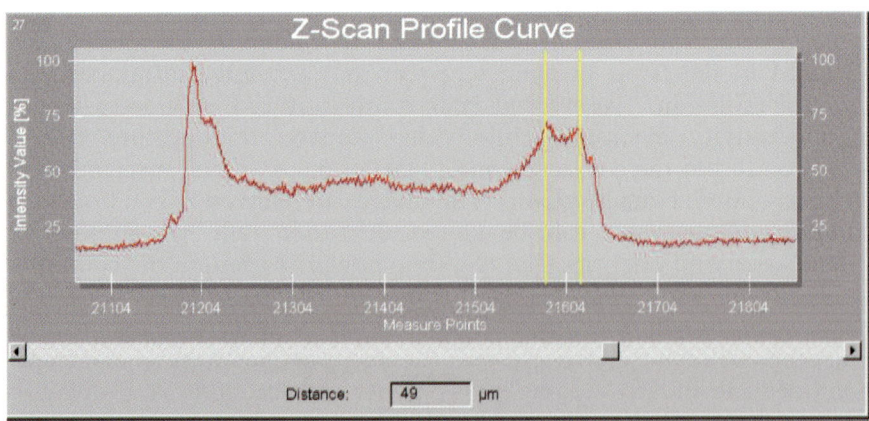

Figure 3.4 Z-scan of a normal human cornea, showing reflected light intensity (*y*-axis) and distance into the cornea (*x*-axis). The peak at left corresponds to the endothelium, and the two peaks corresponding to the yellow line markers at right indicate the anterior and posterior aspects of the epithelium. The epithelium here is 49 μm thick (Courtesy of Maldonado-Codina and O'Donnell, 1999)

anterior and posterior corneal surfaces, and the epithelial–stromal interface, are clearly identifiable as peaks of light intensity on the Z-scan readout. Any opacities in the cornea, or general loss of clarity, will manifest on the Z-scan as an increased intensity. A fundamental limitation of this Z-scan mode is that it does not compensate for movements of the cornea along the anterior–posterior dimension (Z-axis), which are inevitable. That is, there is no fixed depth reference. For this reason, it is necessary to average the information obtained from the multiple scans to determine the depth of any element within the cornea, and such depth information can only be considered to be approximate.

Patient examination

The confocal microscope is housed in a dedicated clinical examination room, and the lights are dimmed prior to the microscopy procedure. To minimize the possibility of cross-contamination between patients, the objective lens is disinfected with isopropyl alcohol before each use. The patient is seated on a comfortable seat behind the instrument and one drop of anaesthetic (benoxinate hydrochloride 0.4%) is instilled into the eye. The head of the patient is placed in the head and chin rest, and the overall height of the instrument table is adjusted for comfort. The patient is instructed to gaze straight ahead; a fixation target is attached to the chin and head rest to facilitate steady fixation.

A large drop of Viscotears® Liquid Gel is applied to the end of the objective lens. The objective lens is brought forwards until the gel comes into contact with the anaesthetized cornea (the objective lens never touches the cornea). As soon as the gel contacts the cornea, the computer monitor displays real-time images. The examination room is arranged in such a way that the operator can see the objective lens on the cornea and the video monitor in the same field of view. The X-controls (side to side) and Y-controls (up and down) are manipulated to align the objective lens with the centre of the cornea; good alignment is confirmed by a bright, even image across the full field, as viewed on the monitor. Image fading towards the edge of the field is occasionally experienced due to non-perfect normal alignment with the cornea and/or natural corneal curvature; this is acceptable as long as the key features of interest are clearly captured. The Z-control (front to back) is dialled back and forth slowly and steadily through the entire corneal thickness. The operator may pause in a particular field of interest (e.g. the anterior and posterior stroma) to effect the capture of a greater number of video frames, thus affording greater flexibility and redundancy with respect to subsequent detailed image analysis. The patient is instructed to sit back and relax while the video image is quickly checked to ensure that the required images have been captured and are of sufficient quality for the intended investigation. If this is satisfactory, the patient is either discharged or repositioned behind the chin and head rest so that the procedure can be repeated on the fellow eye.

From the standpoint of the patient, the procedure is quick and painless. With very little practice, a good-quality single scan from the anterior corneal surface, to the posterior surface and back to the anterior surface takes between 15 and 45 seconds. The patient only needs to be in the confocal microscope examination room for 5 to 10 minutes.

The normal cornea

The structure of the cornea has been described in minute detail as a result of exhaustive studies using light and electron microscopy (see Chapter 4). Nevertheless, it is important to construct a detailed model of the normal cornea as viewed with the confocal microscope so that any suspected corneal abnormalities viewed with this instrument can be discerned.

Population study

In anticipation of an ongoing programme of research centring around the confocal microscope in our laboratory, an extensive qualitative and quantitative evaluation was undertaken of the normal cornea. Images were captured of the central corneas of 50 subjects who were evenly distributed in age from 10 to 80 years.

Qualitative analysis

The epithelium consists of three layers – the superficial cells, wing cells and basal cells. The superficial cell layer is difficult to image with the confocal microscope and is only occasionally seen in some subjects, or when the epithelium has been disturbed (as in contact lens wear). When this layer can be imaged, the superficial cells can be seen to be 40–50 μm in diameter (Figure 3.5). There are large variations in brightness and granularity from cell to cell and within individual cells. Some large dark featureless areas are evident between cells. Small bright rounded nuclei, about 10 μm in diameter, are visible in a small number of cells. The different levels of cytoplasmic reflectivity from cell to cell are thought to represent various stages of progression towards cell death, with the darker cells being those about to desquamate (Wilson, 2000).

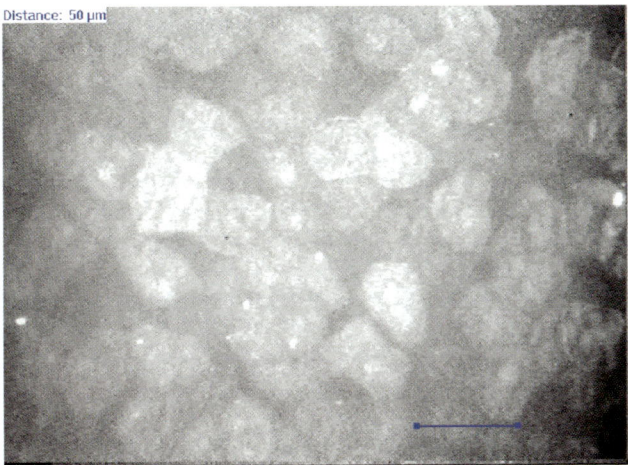

Figure 3.5 Superficial cells of the epithelium

Wing cells are typically 30–45 µm in diameter (Figure 3.6). A very thin border, which is more reflective (brighter) than the cytoplasm, can be seen in many cells. The junction between cells that do not have reflective borders can be deduced from differences in reflectivity of the cytoplasm of adjacent cells. Individual cells are roughly rounded in shape, and have from 5 to 10 sides; some sides are straight and some are curved. As is also evident from specular microscope images of the superficial epithelium, some wing cells appear to have a light grey

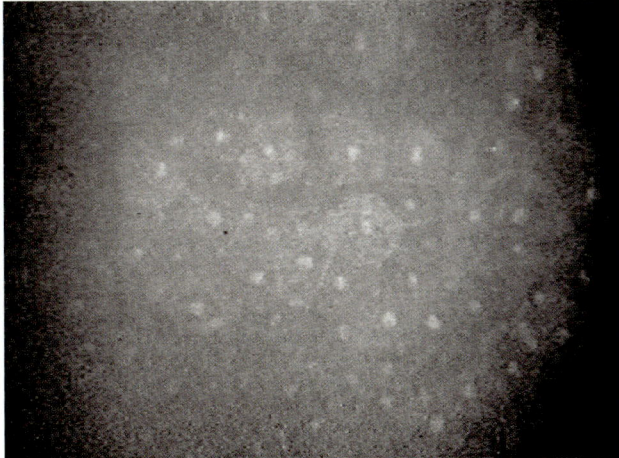

Figure 3.6 Wing cells of the epithelium

cytoplasm and others a dark grey cytoplasm (also referred to as high and low reflectivity), but the variation in reflectivity among wing cells is less marked than that between superficial cells. Small discrete bright nuclei, approximately 5–8 µm in diameter, are visible in the centre of all wing cells.

The basal cells are tightly packed and appear as a uniform field of bright cell borders and dark cytoplasmic mass (Figure 3.7). It is known

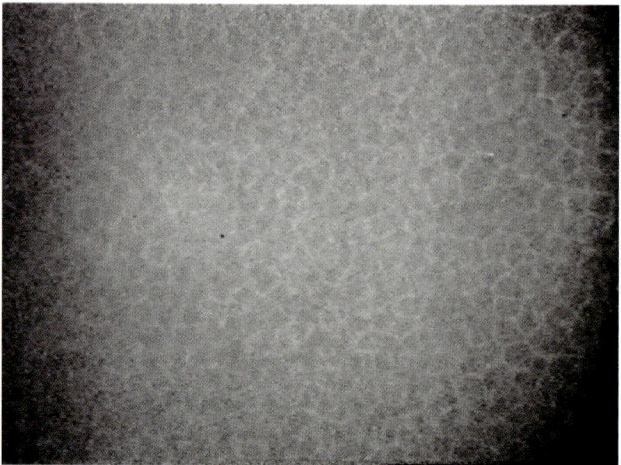

Figure 3.7 Basal cells of the epithelium

from light microscopy that these cells are columnar in shape with the major axis in the anterior–posterior direction (Bron *et al.*, 1997). The confocal view is normal to this axis, which is why the cells appear to be much smaller in diameter (approximately 10 µm) than wing cells or superficial cells. The overall pattern of the basal cell layer is similar to that seen on the side of a giraffe. Cell nuclei are not visible.

The anterior limiting lamina (Bowman's membrane) is known to be amorphous from light and electron microscope studies (Bron *et al.*, 1997). The location of this layer is apparent in the course of focusing through the cornea. After focusing posteriorly through the basal epithelial cell layer, there is a moment when the image becomes featureless and grey, apart from discrete bright beaded nerve fibres of the subepithelial neural plexus that traverse the field of view (Figure 3.8). The odd keratocyte or patch of basal epithelial cells can sometimes be seen in parts of the field if the objective lens deviates from being normal to the corneal surface. The anterior limiting lamina appears somewhat more hazy in older patients.

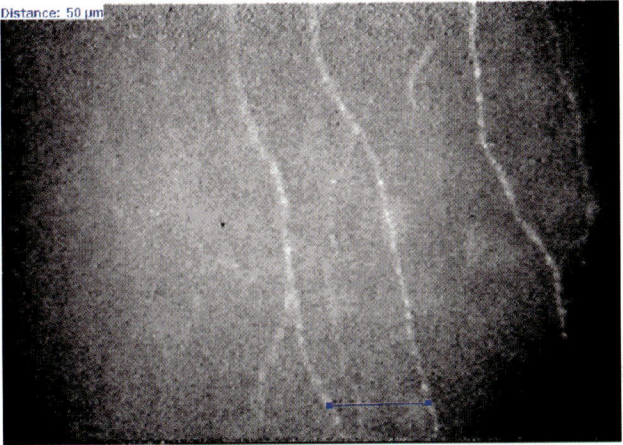

Figure 3.8 The anterior limiting lamina (Bowman's membrane)

The stroma, which accounts for 90% of the thickness of the cornea, is arbitrarily divided into anterior and posterior zones for the purpose of this analysis. Some authors (e.g. Hahnel *et al.*, 2000) prefer to consider the stroma in terms of three zones, considering also the mid-stroma. In reality, there is probably a continuum of change from the anterior to posterior stroma.

The stroma is primarily composed of collagen fibres, ground substance, keratocytes and nerve fibres. The collagen fibres and ground substance cannot be imaged with the confocal microscope, and essentially form the amorphous grey background against which other features are observed. Keratocytes can be identified as discrete bright entities. The cytoplasm, cell walls and processes of keratocytes are not visible; thus, the bright entities are the keratocyte nuclei. In the anterior

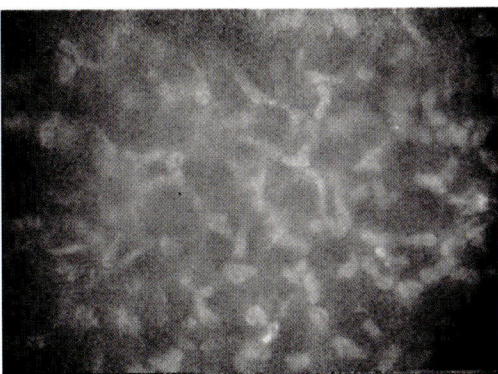

Figure 3.9 The anterior stroma

stroma (Figure 3.9), these nuclei vary from being cigar-shaped to round; this variation in shape can be attributed to different orientations in which the cells are lying in the context of considering the stroma three-dimensionally (Hahnel *et al.*, 2000). There is a commensurate variation in the apparent size of keratocyte nuclei as imaged with the confocal microscope, with their apparent diameter ranging from 5 to 30 μm. Keratocytes in the posterior stroma are less densely packed, and overall the nuclei appear to be slightly larger and flatter (Figure 3.10). A

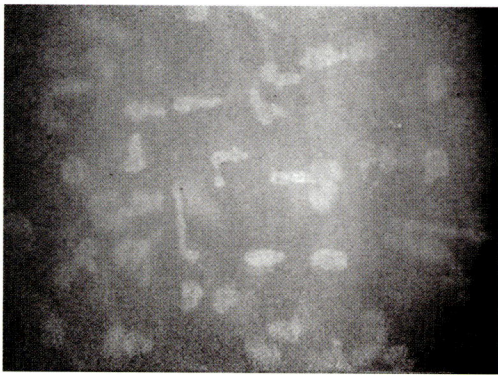

Figure 3.10 The posterior stroma

random array of dark straight lines, termed 'folds', can be observed in the posterior stroma in 10%, 18% and 29% of the population in the fifth, sixth and seventh decades of life, respectively (Figure 3.11). Nerve fibres (Figure 3.12) are occasionally seen traversing the field; these appear slightly thicker and brighter than those seen in the anterior limiting lamina. Other cells known to occasionally populate the stroma, such as monocytes and polymorphonuclear leucocytes, are not observed.

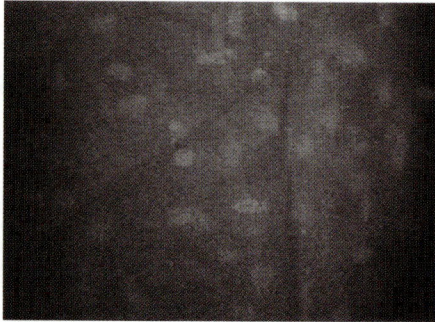

Figure 3.11 Folds in the posterior stroma of a 72-year-old male

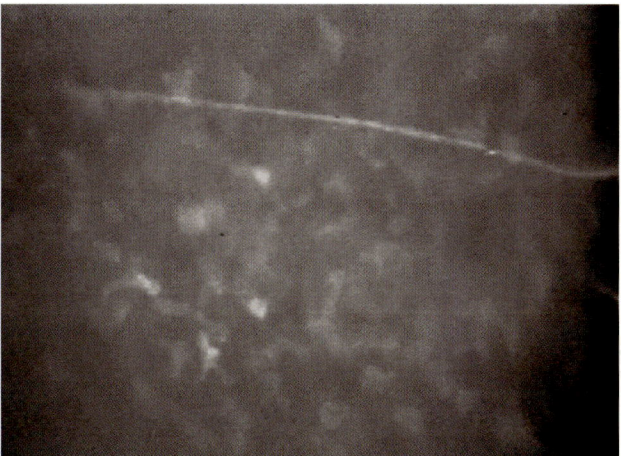

Figure 3.12 Stromal nerve fibre

Small dense highly reflective or 'bright white' dots, about 1–2 μm in diameter – termed 'microdots' by Böhnke and Masters (1997) – can be observed throughout the stroma in virtually all corneas from all age groups, although they appear to be more prevalent in older subjects (Figure 3.13). Because of their ubiquitous nature, microdots must be considered to be a normal feature of human corneal morphology. (This view is contrary to that of Böhnke and Masters (1997), who consider microdots to represent a disease process.) The origin and structural/functional significance of microdots are not known. They may represent dysgenic or apoptotic cellular remnants lying dormant in the stroma (see the section 'Stromal microdots' below on p. 122).

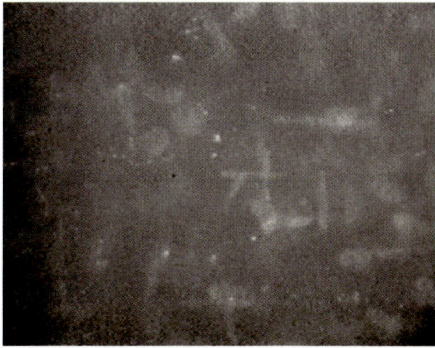

Figure 3.13 Stromal microdots

As with the anterior limiting lamina, the posterior limiting lamina (Descemet's membrane) is featureless and its position can only be deduced in the course of through-focusing from the posterior stroma to the endothelial cells (Figure 3.14). This layer appears to be more granular in elderly patients.

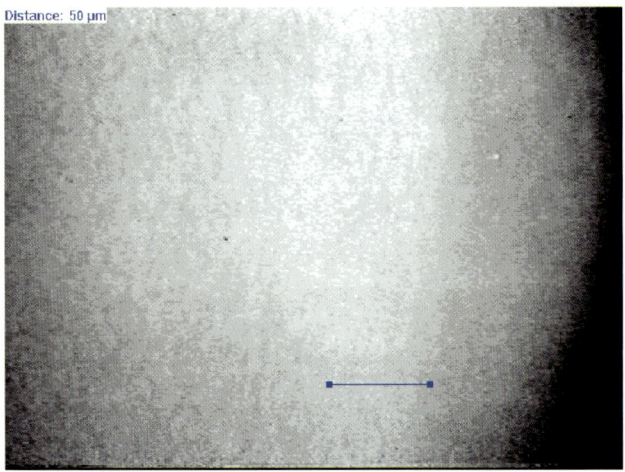

Figure 3.14 The posterior limiting lamina (Descemet's membrane). The anterior surface of some endothelial cells can be seen to the left of the field

The endothelium takes on the classical appearance as seen with specular microscopy (Bron *et al.*, 1997), of an ordered array of primarily five-, six- and seven-sided cells, which have a lightly reflective cytoplasm and clearly defined black cell border (Figure 3.15). It is of interest that this is the opposite polarity of basal epithelial cells, which display a darker cytoplasm and bright border. A slightly darker but very faint nucleus can be observed in a few cells. Endothelial irregularities, presumed to be guttae, are observed in 6%, 12% and 29% of the population in the fifth, sixth and seventh decades of life, respectively (Figure 3.16).

To assist in the interpretation of images of the human cornea using confocal microscopy, a pictorial grid was constructed of the key corneal layers versus age in normal subjects (Perez-Gomez *et al.*, 2000). Images of the central corneas of 119 subjects (age range 11–80 years) were obtained. The clearest image of each corneal layer was selected by one examiner for every subject. These images were grouped together and two examiners selected the most representative image for each corneal

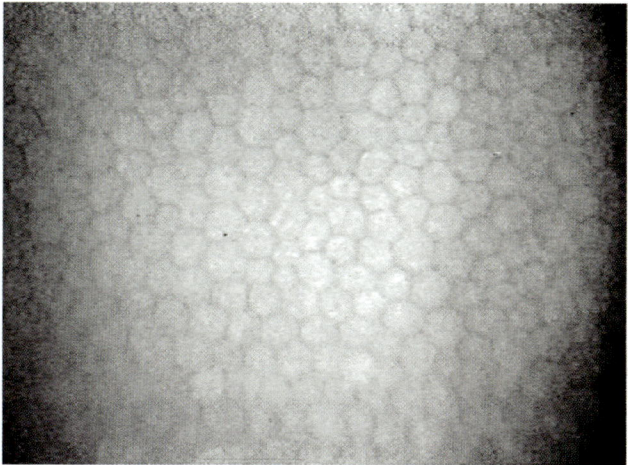

Figure 3.15 The endothelium

layer and decade of life by inspection. These images were then arranged in a grid for ready reference (Figure 3.17). The following features are evident upon inspection of the grid:

1. anterior and posterior keratocyte density decreases with age;
2. endothelial cell density decreases and endothelial polymegethism increases with age;
3. folds appear in the posterior stroma, and guttae appear in the endothelium in the later decades of life.

This grid can assist researchers and clinicians by acting as a normative age-controlled reference against which apparent corneal abnormalities can be assessed.

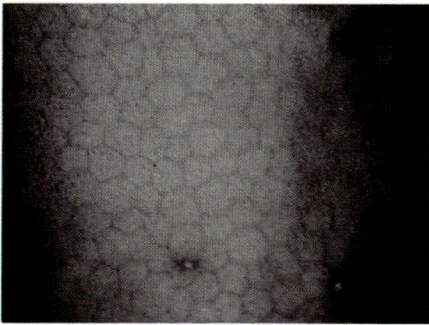

Figure 3.16 Guttae in the endothelium of a 76-year-old female

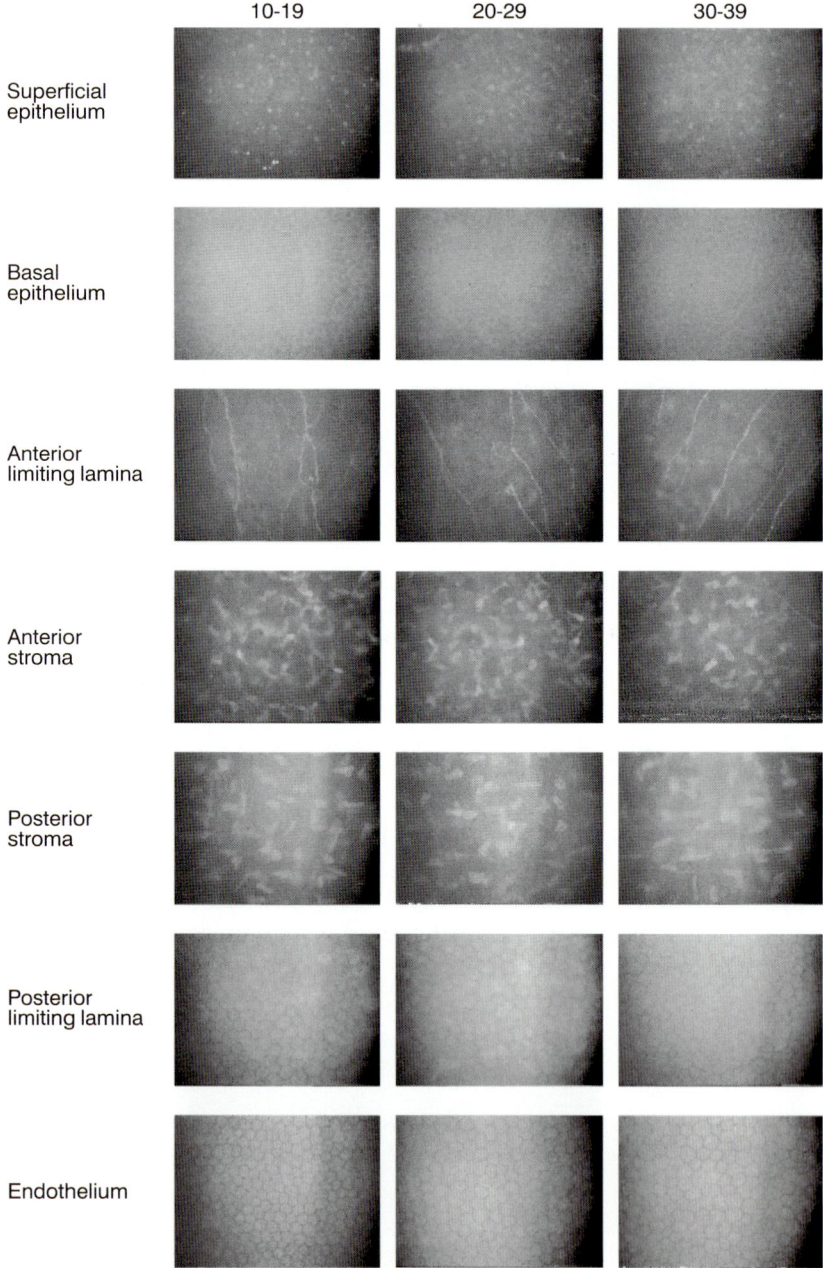

Figure 3.17 Corneal ageing reference grid, depicting changes in the appearance of seven layers of the cornea from the second to the eighth decade of life

40-49 50-59 60-69 70-79

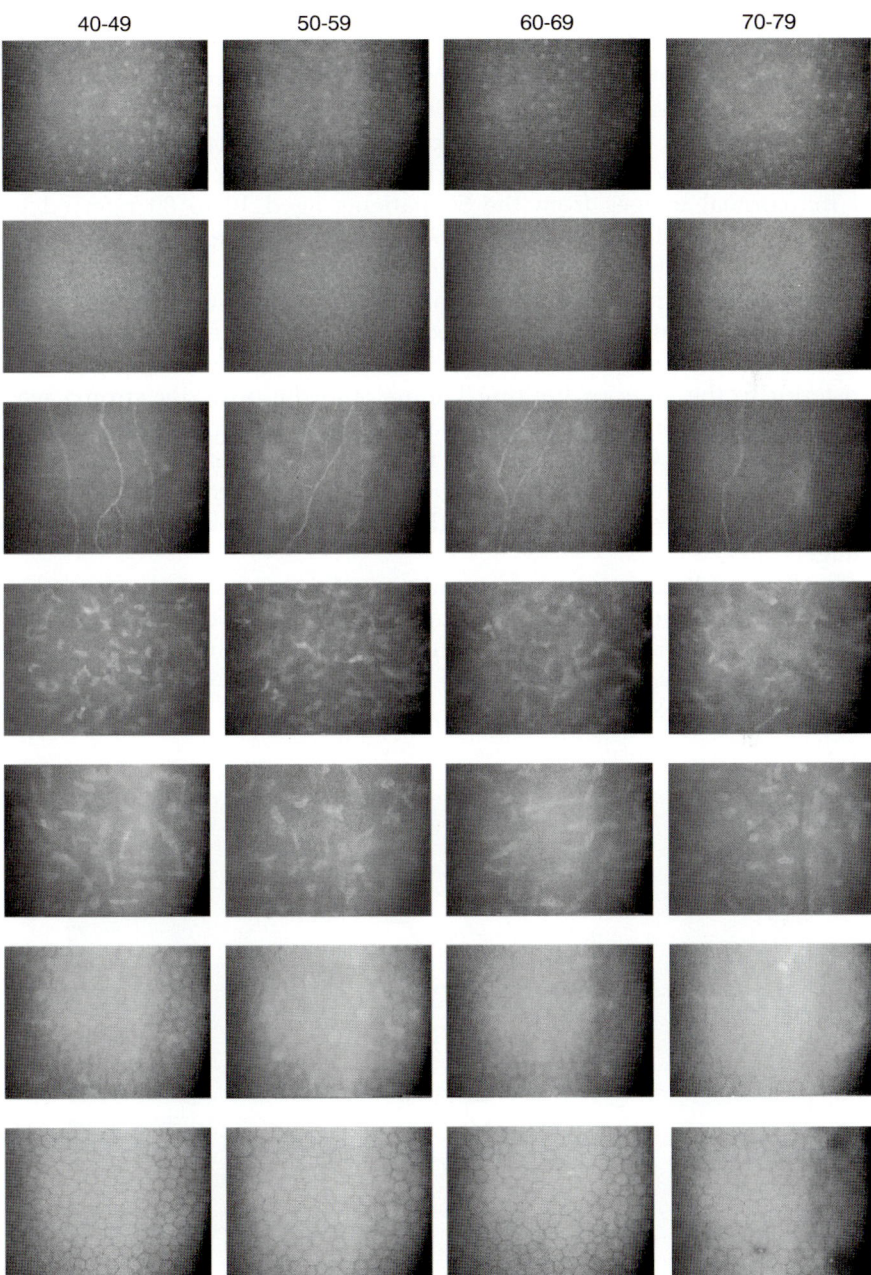

Quantitative analysis

The computer software of the Tomey confocal microscope facilitates manual and semi-automated analysis of any feature of interest. A series of analyses was conducted of epithelial cell morphology, stromal keratocyte density (KCD) and endothelial morphology from some or all of the corneal images from the 50 patients aged 10 to 80 referred to previously (Mutalib *et al.*, 1999). In the first instance, the three best/ clearest images of each of the superficial epithelium, basal epithelium, anterior stroma, posterior stroma and endothelium were selected for each eye of all normal subjects examined. The anterior stroma was taken to be the region of the stroma that came into focus immediately posterior to the anterior limiting lamina, and the posterior stroma was taken to be the region of the stroma that came into focus immediately anterior to the posterior limiting lamina. These images were given random number codes so that the observers conducting the morpho-metric analysis were unaware of the patient age relating to a given image.

Electronic filters were used to enhance the images of the epithelial layers obtained from 13 normal subjects aged 26 ± 4 years. The borders between cells were drawn automatically (Figure 3.18) and the area of individual cells was calculated. The three largest cells in the superficial epithelium and the three smallest cells in the basal epithelium were

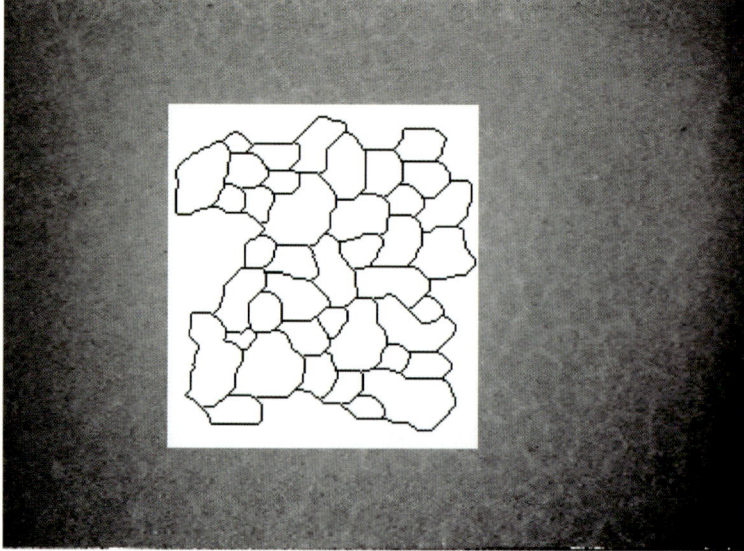

Figure 3.18 The borders of basal epithelial cells identified after application of image enhancement software to a defined region of interest

selected from each image so as to avoid possible misidentification with intermediate-sized wing cells.

The mean area of the superficial and basal cells was 546 ± 51 and $65 \pm 13 \, \mu m^2$, respectively. This compares favourably with the confocal microscopy results of Tomii and Kinoshita (1994), who reported the area of superficial and basal cells to be 624 ± 109 and $66 \pm 5 \, \mu m^2$, respectively. Using specular microscopy, Tsubota and Yamada (1992) found that the area of superficial cells in young adults (26 ± 8 years) was $639 \pm 84 \, \mu m^2$. Although the results of the above three studies were broadly consistent, Mustonen *et al.* (1998), using a scanning slit confocal microscope, reported somewhat higher values of superficial and basal cell areas of 913 ± 326 and $177 \pm 19 \, \mu m^2$, respectively in a slightly older population (45 ± 17 years). The reason for this discrepancy is unclear.

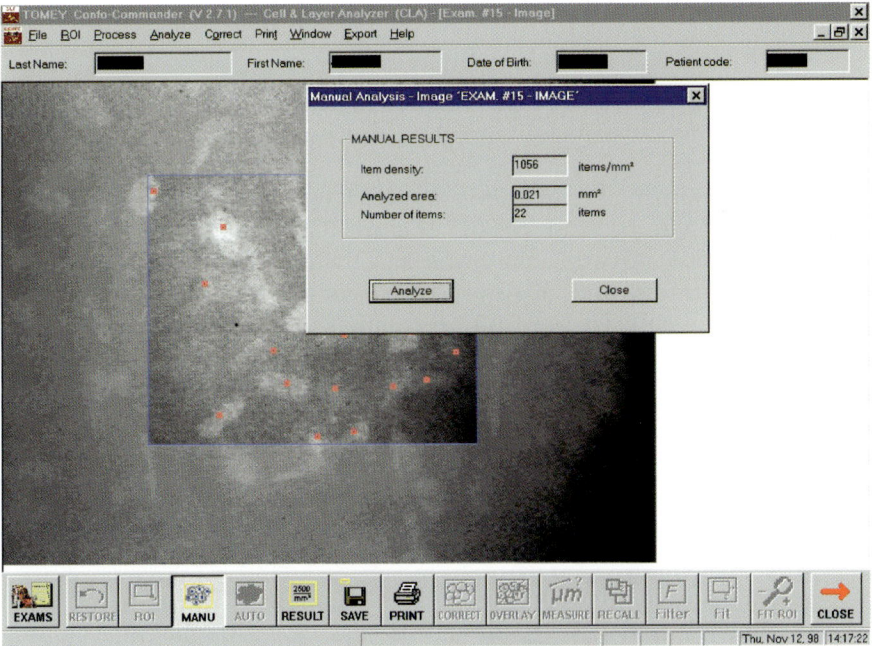

Figure 3.19 Fixed frame technique of analysing keratocyte density in the posterior stroma (Courtesy of Maldonado-Codina and O'Donnell, 1999)

A semi-automated fixed frame technique was used to determine KCD (Figure 3.19). A rectangle of known size ($159 \times 131 \, \mu m$) was electronically interposed onto an image and 'whole' keratocyte nuclei with clearly defined borders were electronically tagged. Keratocyte nuclei overlapping the inferior and left borders of the rectangle were also

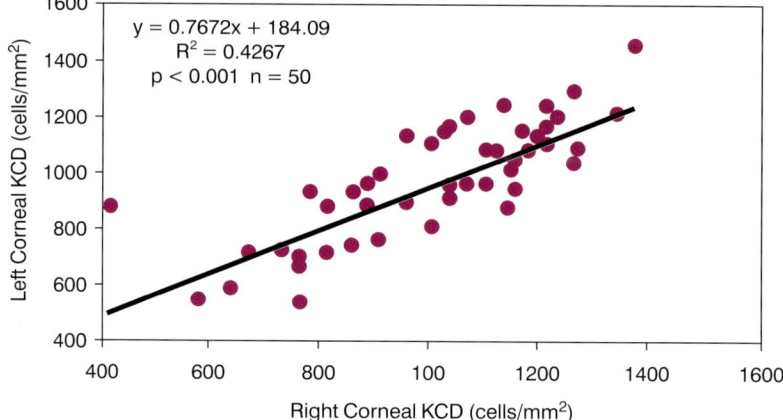

Figure 3.20 Interocular correlation of keratocyte density (KCD) in the anterior stroma

marked. When this task was completed, the computer counted the number of keratocyte nuclei (and thus, the number of keratocytes) per square millimetre visible in the field.

A strong interocular correlation in KCD was observed for both the anterior stroma ($r = 0.81$, $P < 0.001$) (Figure 3.20) and posterior stroma ($r = 0.38$, $P < 0.006$). Overall, the mean KCD was 992 ± 210 cells/mm² for the anterior stroma and 573 ± 61 cells/mm² for the posterior stroma (Mutalib *et al.*, 1999). These results are similar to those of Mustonen *et al.* (1998), who reported KCD in a normal human population to be 1058 ± 217 cells/mm² and 771 ± 135 cells/mm² for the anterior and posterior stroma

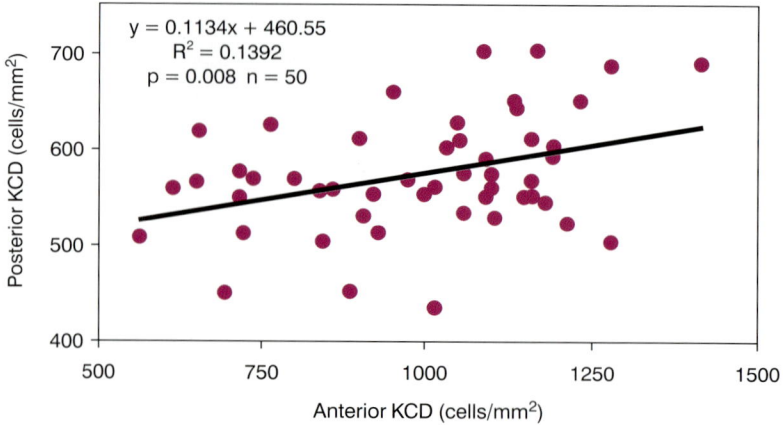

Figure 3.21 Relation between posterior and anterior stromal keratocyte density (KCD)

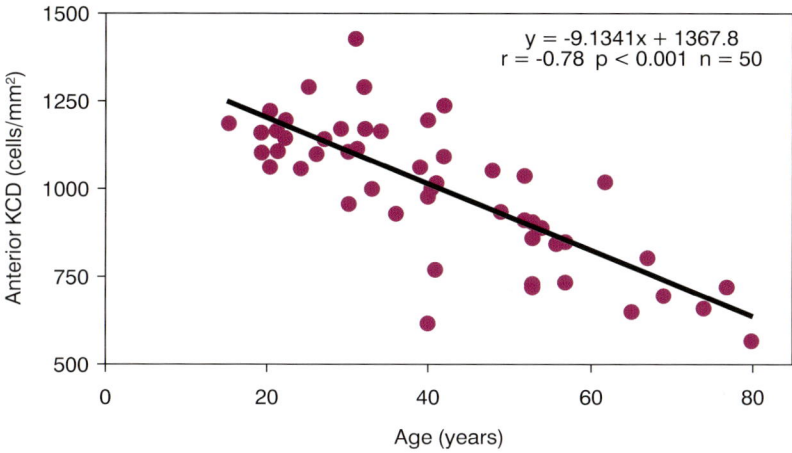

Figure 3.22 Relation between anterior stromal keratocyte density (KCD) and age

respectively. There was a strong correlation between anterior stromal KCD versus posterior stromal KCD (Mutalib *et al.*, 1999) (Figure 3.21).

Anterior stromal KCD was found to decrease throughout life at a rate of 0.1% per year ($r = -0.78$, $P < 0.001$) (Figure 3.22). This decline was apparently less rapid for the posterior stroma (0.01% per year; $r = -0.30$, $P < 0.034$) (Mutalib *et al.*, 1999) (Figure 3.23). Mustonen *et al.* (1998) were unable to detect a change in keratocyte density with age. However, Moller-Pederson (1997) found that stromal DNA in the human cornea decreased throughout life at a rate of 0.3% per year. Since the living cell

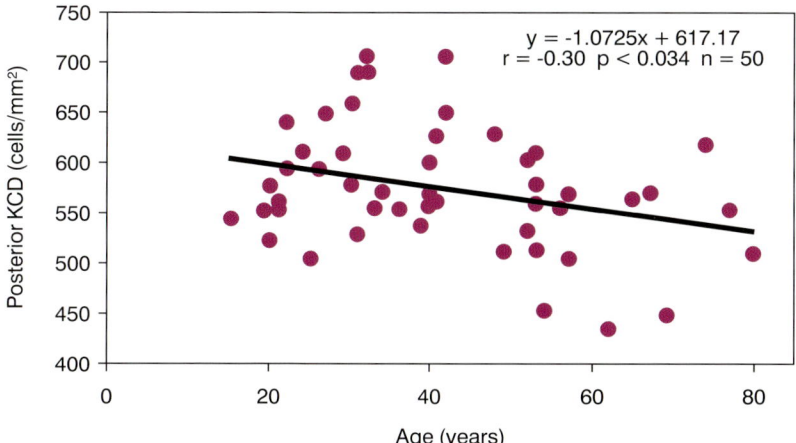

Figure 3.23 Relation between posterior stromal keratocyte density (KCD) and age

population of the stroma consists almost entirely of keratocytes, this decline is likely to reflect a reduction in the total mass of stromal keratocytes. Certainly, a reduction in KCD is consistent with known biochemical changes (Malik *et al.*, 1992) and structural alterations (Olsen and Ehlers, 1984; Malik *et al.*, 1992) to the corneal stroma throughout life.

Endothelial morphology was assessed using the fully automated endothelial analysis software of the Tomey ConfoScan. A suitable image of the endothelium is digitized and a square region of interest is electronically interposed onto the frame. The image is automatically enhanced to sharpen the cell borders, which are electronically traced. Any gaps can be corrected manually. Various parameters are then calculated, including endothelial cell density (ECD) and the coefficient of variation of endothelial cell size (COV; standard deviation of cell area divided by mean cell area), etc. (Figure 3.24).

Endothelial cell density (ECD) was found to be strongly correlated between eyes ($r = 0.68$, $P < 0.001$) (Figure 3.25), and to decrease throughout life at a rate of 0.1% per year ($r = -0.55$, $P < 0.001$) (Figure 3.26) (Mutalib *et al.*, 1999). Mustonen *et al.* (1998) also detected a loss of ECD

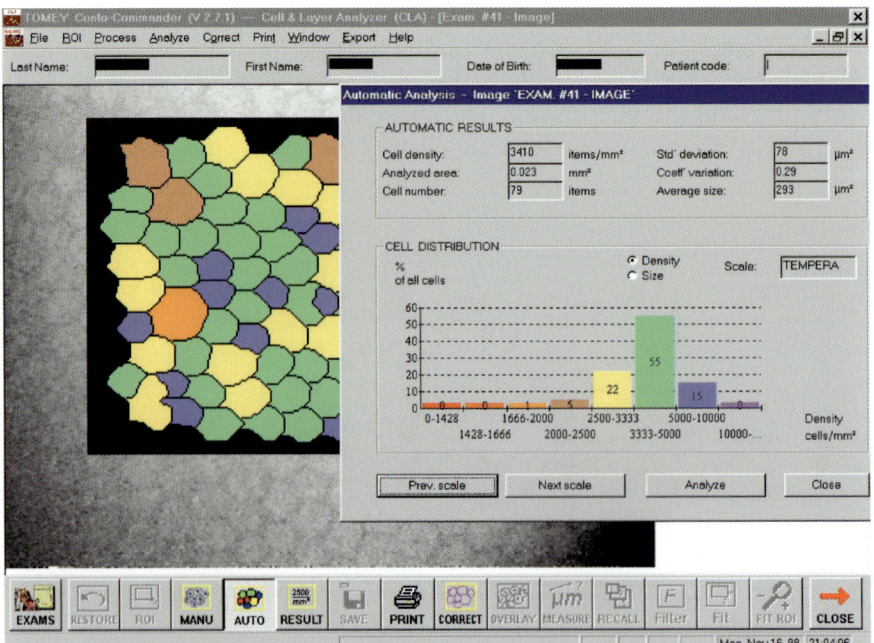

Figure 3.24 Automated analysis of endothelial morphology (Courtesy of Maldonado-Codina and O'Donnell, 1999)

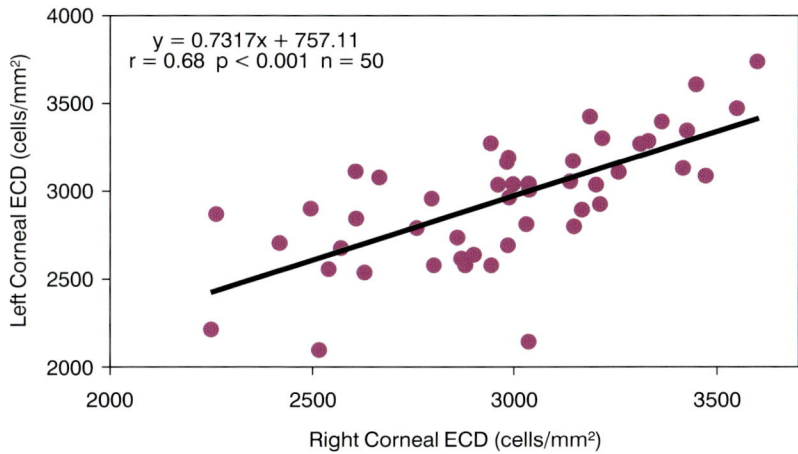

Figure 3.25 Interocular correlation of endothelial cell density (ECD)

with age. The mean COV increased throughout life ($r = 0.37$, $P < 0.008$) (Figure 3.27), which is in agreement with previous work (Bourne *et al.*, 1996).

A significant positive correlation was demonstrated between anterior KCD and ECD ($r = 0.48$; $P < 0.001$) (Mutalib *et al.*, 1999) (Figure 3.28); however, there was no such relationship between posterior KCD and ECD. The significance of the relationship between anterior KCD and ECD is unclear. Moller-Pederson (1997) found a positive correlation between

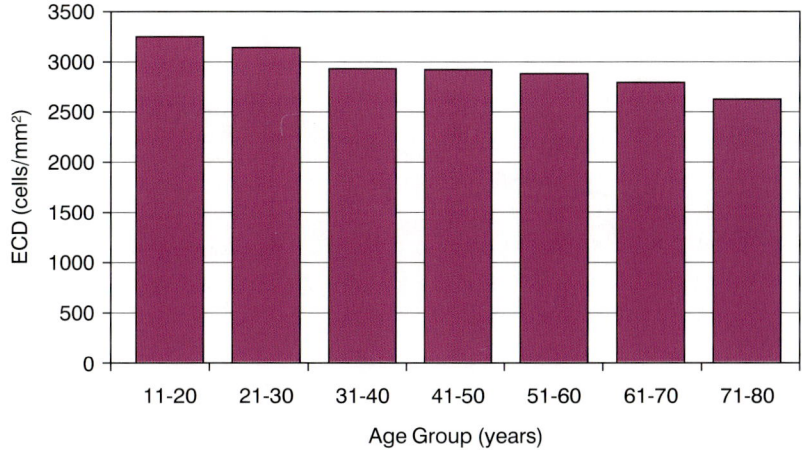

Figure 3.26 Endothelial cell density (ECD) grouped by age decade

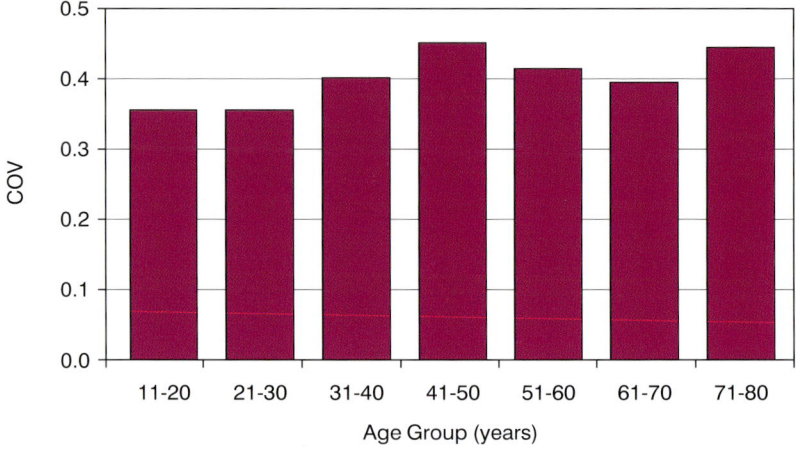

Figure 3.27 Coefficient of endothelial cell size (COV) grouped by age decade

stromal DNA and ECD and suggested that these cell populations may have a similar embryonic origin; however, this may be a casual association due to an age-related decline in anterior KCD and ECD.

Having established qualitative and quantitative population norms relating to the appearance of the human cornea as viewed with the confocal microscope, this technique can be used to assess the effects of contact lens wear on the cornea. A series of preliminary experiments and observations relating to these effects is described below.

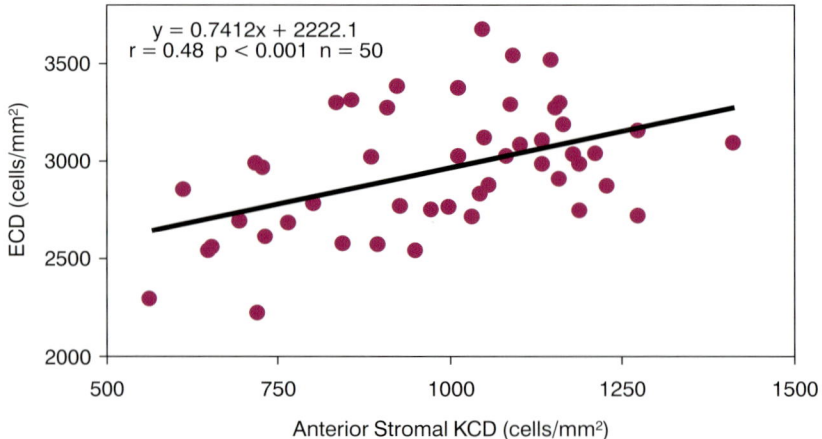

Figure 3.28 Relation between endothelial cell density (ECD) versus anterior stromal keratocyte density (KCD)

The cornea during contact lens wear

The availability of the confocal microscope introduces the prospect of solving problems that have been difficult to investigate due to a lack of resolution and magnification available with existing instruments – primarily the slit lamp. Specifically, it will allow researchers and clinicians to:

1. discover, or understand better, the reason for the appearance of certain phenomena (e.g. stromal striae and folds);
2. verify the pathophysiology of certain conditions that are already thought to be reasonably well understood (e.g. endothelial blebs);
3. make new discoveries relating to corneal features that previously could not be seen (e.g. keratocyte density and stromal microdots).

This section will provide insights into research efforts that have been initiated in order to exploit the potential for the confocal microscope to confirm and/or unravel various manifestations of the ocular response to contact lens wear.

Epithelial cell morphology

Contact lenses protect the surface of the cornea from the normal shearing forces of the eyelids, thus inhibiting cell shedding (Lemp and Mathers, 1989). As a result, it could be expected that there would be evidence of delayed cell desquamation on the epithelial surface of contact lens wearers. Bansal *et al.* (1997) used slit scanning confocal microscopy to compare the epithelium of 20 contact lens wearers versus 36 non-lens-wearing control subjects. They observed that superficial bright epithelial cells were reduced in number in the contact lens wearing group (446 ± 310 cells/mm^2) as compared to the control group (620 ± 210 cells/mm^2).

Using specular microscopy, Tsubota and Yamada (1992) found the size of superficial epithelial cells to increase from $639 \pm 84 \, \mu m^2$ at baseline to $820 \pm 99 \, \mu m^2$ after three months of soft lens wear. They attributed this finding to delayed epithelial desquamation due to contact lens wear. O'Leary *et al.* (1998) employed a corneal irrigation technique to wash desquamated epithelial cells from the surface of the cornea; they observed that desquamated epithelial cells were larger in contact lens wearers ($1436 \, \mu m^2$) versus non-lens wearers ($1225 \, \mu m^2$). The reason for the larger size of desquamated cells may relate to their hypermature status. Jalbert *et al.* (2000) applied both of the techniques used by Tsubota and Yamada (1992) and O'Leary *et al.* (1998), and verified that the cell size values are larger when determined using the irrigation chamber technique than those determined using confocal microscopy.

Bansal *et al.* (1997) found no differences in the number of basal epithelial cells between contact lens wearers and matched controls using confocal microscopy. They also reported that the total axon length of the subepithelial nerve plexus was reduced in soft lens wearers (versus matched controls); however, Oliveira-Soto (1999) attributes apparent changes in nerve morphology observed in contact lens wearers to an artefact due to lens-induced oedema.

Corneal oedema

The human cornea swells by about 4% in thickness during eye closure overnight; it then deswells rapidly following eye opening in the morning (Kiely *et al.*, 1982). The cornea then continues to deswell very slowly (at a rate of 1 μm/h) throughout the waking hours (Kiely *et al.*, 1982). This swelling and deswelling is known to directly reflect changes in corneal hydration because the cornea can only change thickness in the anterior–posterior axis. Thus, a 4% increase in corneal thickness represents a 4% increase in stromal water content, or 4% oedema.

The prevalence of contact lens-induced oedema is essentially 100%, since all contact lenses induce some level of oedema, with the possible exception of silicone elastomer lenses (LaHood *et al.*, 1988). The amount of oedema is related primarily to the extent of corneal hypoxia that is induced by the lens. With current generation soft and rigid lenses, daytime corneal oedema typically varies between 1 and 5%, which in the acute sense can be considered as being safe. The level of overnight oedema measured upon waking generally falls in the range 5–15% (Holden *et al.*, 1983).

Clinicians can estimate the magnitude of corneal oedema via careful observation with the slit lamp, as a number of structural changes can be identified that correlate with various levels of oedema (Efron, 1999). These structural changes – striae, folds and haze – act as useful reference points or 'yardsticks' to form the basis of clinical decision-making (Figure 3.29). When viewed using direct focal illumination, striae appear as fine wispy white vertically oriented lines, and are always located in the posterior stroma (Sarver, 1971) (Figure 3.29). They can also appear as dark lines against the orange fundus pupillary reflex when observed using retro-illumination. Striae are only observed when the level of oedema reaches about 5%, and clinicians are advised to adopt a cautious approach when striae are observed. As the level of oedema increases, striae become greyer and thicker, and they increase in number. Striae do not cause vision loss.

Folds can be observed in the endothelial mosaic as a combination of depressed grooves or raised ridges, or as a general area of apparent buckling (Figure 3.29), when the level of oedema reaches about 8%. They

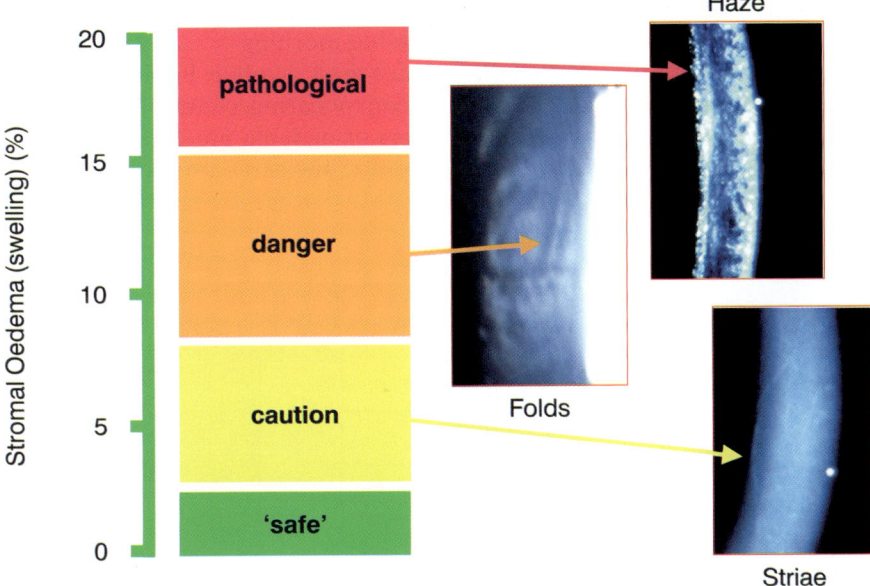

Figure 3.29 Signs of various levels of oedema observed using a slit lamp

also increase in number as the level of oedema increases (LaHood and Grant, 1990). Folds are best observed using specular reflection. Vision is thought to be unaffected by folds; nevertheless, clinicians should consider this to be a 'danger sign', especially if observed in patients using daily wear lenses.

The stroma takes on a hazy, milky or granular appearance when the level of oedema reaches about 15% (Figure 3.29). In essence, the stroma has suffered a loss of transparency, and is essentially in a pathological state. This condition can be viewed using a variety of observation techniques. The milky appearance is evident when the cornea is viewed against the pupil using indirect illumination. Instead of the normal dark appearance, a fine grey haze is detected and fine iris detail is partially obscured. Sclerotic scatter technique will enhance this clinical picture. Contact lens-induced stromal haze can cause a slight degradation of vision when the level of oedema exceeds 20%.

An experiment was conducted so that oedematous corneal changes could be examined using confocal microscopy (Efron *et al.*, 1999). Thirteen human subjects participated; these comprised 10 females and 3 males, aged 24 ± 3 years. Three subjects had worn contact lenses previously. Each subject was fitted with a -3.00 D soft contact lens of Dk/t of 15.1×10^{-9} (cm/ s) $\times$ (ml O_2/ml $\times$ mmHg), which was worn in one eye only during sleep for 8 hours overnight. Confocal microscopy, slit lamp biomicroscopy and ultrasonic pachometry were performed on both eyes before lens insertion at night and after lens removal the following morning.

Pachometry confirmed that the cornea had swollen by 11.8% in the lens-wearing eye and 2.1% in the non-lens-wearing control eye ($P < 0.01$ for both eyes) (Figure 3.30). These levels of oedema are consistent with those observed in previous studies adopting the same protocol (LaHood

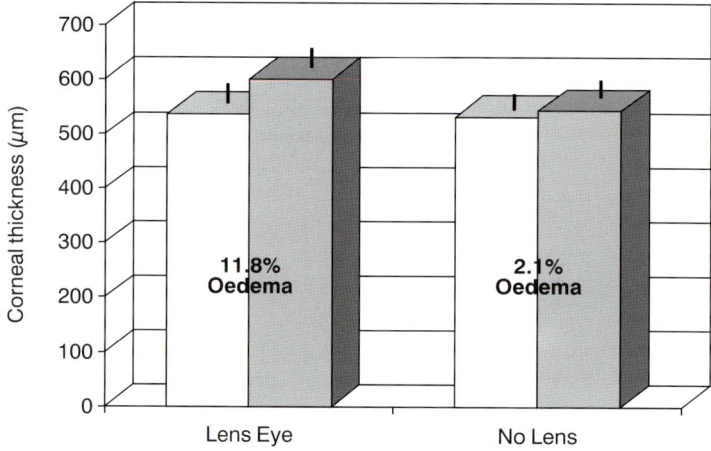

Figure 3.30 Corneal thickness before sleep (white bars) and after sleep (grey bars) in the lens-wearing eyes (left) and non-lens-wearing control eyes (right)

et al., 1988). Striae and folds were observed in the lens-wearing eyes with the slit lamp (Figure 3.31). With the confocal microscope, long dark lines could be observed in the posterior stroma of the lens-wearing eyes (Figure 3.31). These lines were orthogonal and generally oriented horizontally and vertically. The prevalence of these lines varied throughout the depth of the posterior stroma. The thickness of the lines, and the total number of lines observed, was greater at higher levels of oedema.

To facilitate analysis of corneal oedema as viewed with the confocal microscope, a grading scale was constructed (Figure 3.32); this depicts images of the basal epithelium, anterior and posterior stroma and endothelium at baseline (0% oedema) and four levels of swelling (Mutalib and Efron, 1999):

Grade 1: 1–4%
Grade 2: 5–7%
Grade 3: 8–14%
Grade 4: >14% oedema

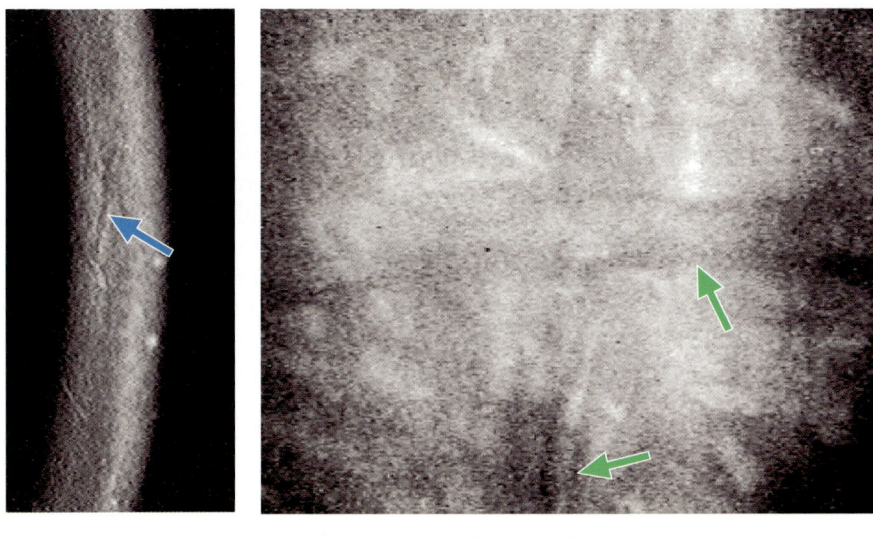

Slit Lamp   Confocal Microscope

Figure 3.31 Left: Dark vertical furrows observed in the posterior stroma using the slit lamp (blue arrow). Right: Dark horizontal and vertical lines observed in the posterior stroma (green arrows) of the same patient

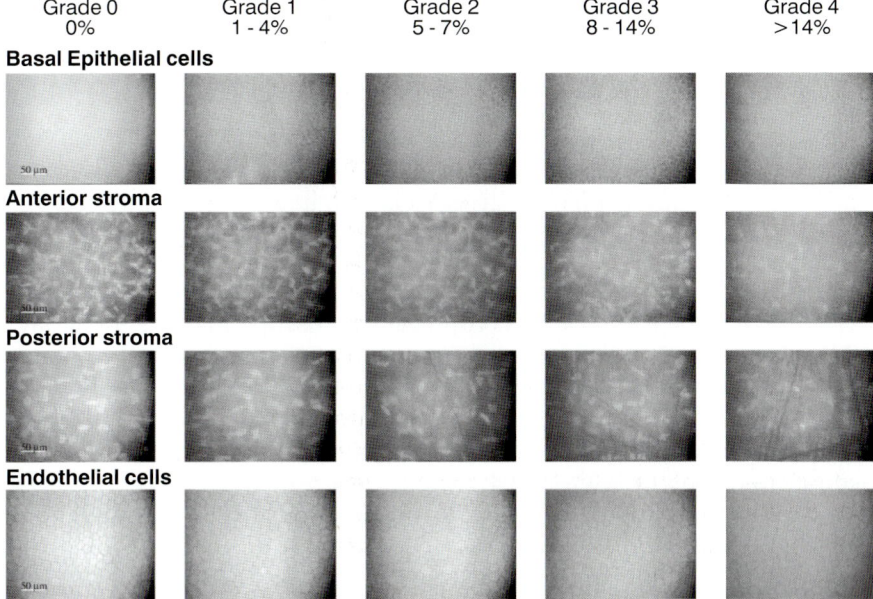

Figure 3.32 Grading scales for assessing the effects of oedema on the basal epithelium, anterior and posterior stroma and endothelium using the confocal microscope. The corresponding percentage stromal oedema is indicated below each grade caption

Features of the basal epithelium become more distinct at higher levels of oedema due to greater contrast whereby the borders appear brighter and the cytoplasm darker. In the anterior stroma, the keratocyte nuclei become less distinct and apparently fewer in number at higher levels of oedema. A similar trend is noted in the posterior stroma, which in addition can be seen to have a lower overall cell density compared with the anterior stroma. Dark lines begin to appear at about 5–7% oedema, and a positive correlation was found to exist between the level of corneal oedema and the severity of folds ($r = 0.94$, $P < 0.001$) (Mutalib and Efron, 1999) (Figure 3.33). The endothelial mosaic becomes less distinct at higher levels of oedema.

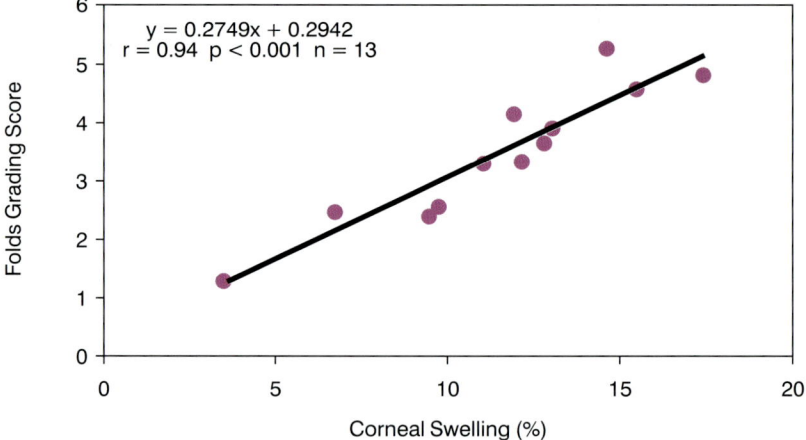

Figure 3.33 Relationship between corneal oedema and the severity of folds in the posterior stroma as viewed with the confocal microscope

The dark lines seen with the confocal microscope and the striae and folds seen with the slit lamp are likely to be different optical views of the same phenomena. Certainly, the relationship between the level of oedema and the number of folds as determined by LaHood and Grant (1990) is almost identical to the relationship between the level of oedema and the grading of dark lines as determined in this work using the confocal microscope (Mutalib and Efron, 1999) (Figure 3.33). However, there are some anomalies. Striae, as distinct from folds, are not seen with the confocal microscope. Images obtained with the confocal microscope suggest that striae and folds are essentially a continuum of the same process, but perhaps observed at different stages of formation. That is, striae seen with the slit lamp and fine black lines seen with the confocal microscope at around 5% oedema are probably the same entity. Similarly, folds seen with the slit lamp may be the equivalent of heavy black lines seen with the confocal microscope at around 10% oedema.

Clinicians have long been unclear as to why striae, and to a lesser degree folds, almost always appear to be vertically oriented (Sarver, 1971). Certainly, the dark lines observed in the oedematous cornea with the confocal microscope appear in both vertical and horizontal orientations. Some researchers believe that the appearance of vertical striae may be related to the vertical orientation of the slit lamp illumination beam; however, the slit aperture in the confocal microscope is also vertically oriented. Perhaps the horizontally displaced eyepieces used to obtain a binocular view with the slit lamp preclude the visualization of horizontal striae with this instrument. Further experiments using the slit lamp, in which these oedematous formations are viewed with the eye, the slit illumination and the binocular objectives at different orthogonal angles, may provide the answer to this dilemma.

Quantitative analysis of stromal keratocyte populations before and after sleep revealed that keratocyte density had apparently dropped overnight by 21% and 20% in the anterior and posterior stroma of the lens-wearing eye, and by 11% and 9% in the anterior and posterior stroma of the non-lens-wearing eye; these differences were statistically significant (Figure 3.34) (P <0.001). It is unlikely that such a dramatic shift in the stromal keratocyte population reflects a diurnal cycle of cell death and regeneration, and an alternative explanation must be sought.

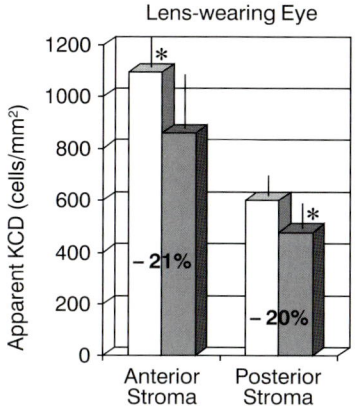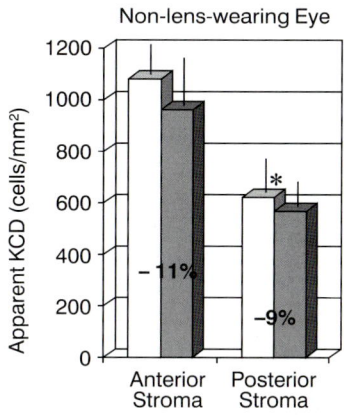

Figure 3.34 Keratocyte density before sleep (white bars) and after sleep (grey bars) in the anterior and posterior stroma of the lens-wearing eyes (left frame) and non-lens-wearing control eyes (right frame). Error bars represent +1 standard deviation and the asterisks indicate statistical significance of the difference between the adjacent bars

A simple geometric model can be constructed to help explain this observation. In Figure 3.35, the section of stromal tissue at left contains a fixed number of keratocytes. When viewed with the confocal microscope, only those keratocytes located within a 10 μm deep slice of tissue (equivalent to the depth of field of the confocal microscope) can be seen. Assume that the cornea has become swollen, and the total number of keratocytes remains the same. In fact, the stroma has become elongated along a single anterior–posterior axis, which is the only dimension in which the human cornea can swell (Figure 3.35 right). The keratocytes are now more spread out within this tissue section. Since the depth of field of

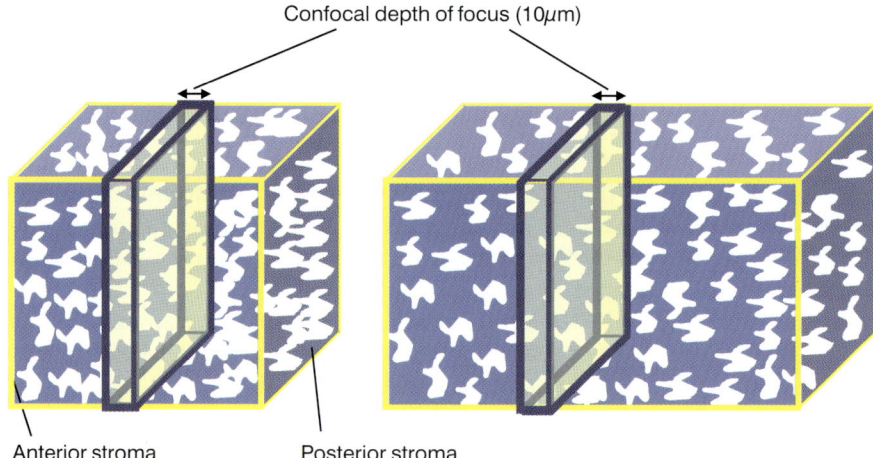

Confocal depth of focus (10μm)

Anterior stroma   Posterior stroma

Figure 3.35 Left: Stromal keratocytes (white) can be seen in the 10 μm thick section (yellow) of stromal tissue (blue) with the confocal microscope. Right: The stromal tissue has become swollen and expanded in one dimension (along the anterior–posterior axis). Assuming that the number of keratocytes has remained constant, fewer keratocytes will be seen in the 10 μm thick swollen section with the confocal microscope, giving rise to the illusion of a reduction in the number of keratocytes

the confocal microscope remains the same, fewer keratocytes can be seen in a 10 μm slice of tissue, giving the false impression of a loss of keratocytes.

A binomial expansion model suggests that the magnitude of the apparent loss of keratocytes should be roughly equivalent to the level of oedema. However, taking the lens-wearing eye as an example, the percentage loss of keratocytes (21% and 20% in the anterior and posterior stroma, respectively) is far greater than the percentage increase on overnight corneal oedema (11.8%). The reason for this discrepancy probably relates to the fact that the confocal images of stromal tissue become dramatically less distinct as the stroma swells, as can be seen from Figure 3.32. Keratocyte nuclei are less easy to see, and therefore count, in the presence of high levels of oedema. Thus, the apparent drop in KCD in the oedematous cornea is likely to be an artefact that can be explained in terms of (1) unidimensional volumetric stromal expansion viewed with a confocal microscope that has a fixed depth of focus, and (2) a degradation of image quality at higher levels of oedema making keratocytes more difficult to detect. Of course, this observation could also be explained by a real loss of keratocytes; however, a large diurnal cycle of keratocyte death overnight and regeneration during the day is unlikely.

Stromal keratocyte density

In 1985, Holden and co-workers reported that long-term contact lens wear causes stromal thinning (Holden *et al.*, 1985a). Specifically, they demonstrated that the central stroma of 27 patients had thinned by an average of 11 µm (2.3%) after five years of extended wear of 71% water content lenses. These authors suggested that thinning could be due to chronic adverse effects of oedema and/or hypoxia on the integrity of keratocytes, which are known to be responsible for synthesizing the bulk of the collagen, glycoproteins and proteoglycans in the stroma. More recently, Liu and Pflugfelder (2000) reported 30–50 µm thinning in the central and peripheral cornea of 35 patients who had worn contact lenses for an average of 6.4 years. However, contact lens wear is also known to induce thinning of the corneal epithelium, so the amount of stromal thinning reported in the study of Liu and Pflugfelder (2000) may have been less than 30–50 µm. This would be more consistent with the results of Holden *et al.* (1985a).

Jalbert and Stapleton (1999) used the confocal microscope to measure KCD in nine subjects wearing disposable hydrogel lenses and nine age- and sex-matched non-lens-wearing control subjects. They reported that KCD was reduced in the lens-wearing group in both the anterior stroma (544 ± 206 cells/mm^2 versus 804 ± 145 cells/mm^2 in the non-lens-wearing group) ($P < 0.01$) and posterior stroma (514 ± 111 cells/mm^2 versus 628 ± 101 cells/mm^2 in the non-lens-wearing group) ($P < 0.05$). Jalbert and Stapleton (1999) concluded that their findings indicate that extended wear of hydrogel lenses reduces stromal keratocyte density, which was perhaps due to hypoxic, cytokine-mediated or mechanical effects. Bansal *et al.* (1997) also reported that anterior KCD in contact lens wearers (757 ± 243 cells/mm^2) was significantly less than that in normals (925 ± 276 cells/mm^2).

The loss of keratocytes reported by Jalbert and Stapleton (1999) and Bansal *et al.* (1997) could be partially attributable to an artefact relating to the presence of residual oedema in the cornea at the time of undertaking confocal microscopy, as explained above. Although these authors did remove the contact lenses prior to measuring corneal thickness, Holden *et al.* (1985a) have previously demonstrated that chronic lens-induced oedema can take up to 7 days to dissipate.

To explore this phenomenon further, Morgan *et al.* (2000) conducted a prospective study of the effects of lens wear on KCD that was designed to account for the oedema effect discussed above. A group of 23 subjects, who had never before worn contact lenses ('neophytes'), were fitted with a PureVision lens (Bausch & Lomb) and the Acuvue 2 lens (Vistakon) on a contralateral basis (Table 3.1). Corneal thickness was measured using

Table 3.1 Lenses used by Morgan *et al.* (2000)		
	PureVision	*Acuvue 2*
Manufacturer	Bausch & Lomb	Vistakon, Johnson & Johnson
Material	Balafilcon A	Etafilcon A
*Dk**	99	28
Nominal water content	36%	58%

$* \times 10^{-11}$ (cm^2/s) (ml O$_2$/ml $\times$ mmHg)

ultrasonic pachometry and KCD was determined with the confocal microscope; these assessments were conducted at baseline (before lens wear), after six months of lens wear, and one week after ceasing lens wear.

As expected, corneal thickness was different for the two lenses overall ($F = 7.4$, $P = 0.0079$). Inspection of Figure 3.36 indicates that corneal thickness was similar for the two lenses at the initial and final visits, but was greater for the Acuvue 2 lens at the six-month visit. Indeed, these corneal thickness changes were consistent with the relative oxygen performances of the two lens types. Corneal thickness with the Acuvue 2 lens was about 2% greater at the six-month visit than at the initial visit, whereas there was no change with the PureVision lens.

No differences were established between the two lenses ($F = 2.5$, $P = 0.1174$) or the three study visits ($F = 0.9$, $P = 0.4276$) for anterior stromal KCD. Posterior stromal KCD was similar for the two lenses throughout the study ($F = 0.2$, $P = 0.6723$); however, there were differences between

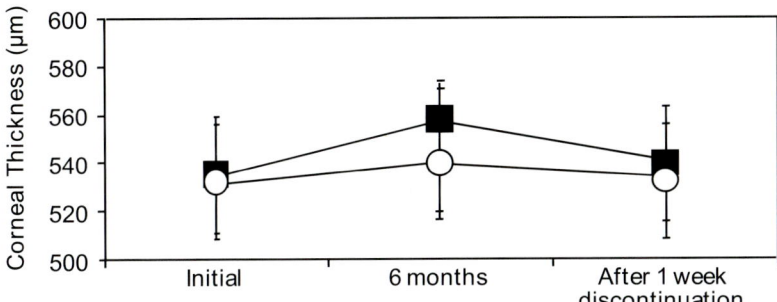

Figure 3.36 Corneal thickness (μm) before lens wear (initial), after six months of wear, and one week after discontinuing lens wear in eyes wearing a PureVision lens (white circles) and an Acuvue 2 lens (black squares). Error bars represent ±1 standard deviation

the three visits ($F = 13.8$, $P = 0.0001$). Post hoc analysis confirmed that the cell counts at the six-month and final visits, were lower than at the initial visit (Figure 3.37).

The 14% reduction in posterior stromal KCD with the extended wear of soft lenses reported in the study of Morgan *et al.* (2000) therefore confirms the earlier observations of Jalbert and Stapleton (1999) and Bansal *et al.*

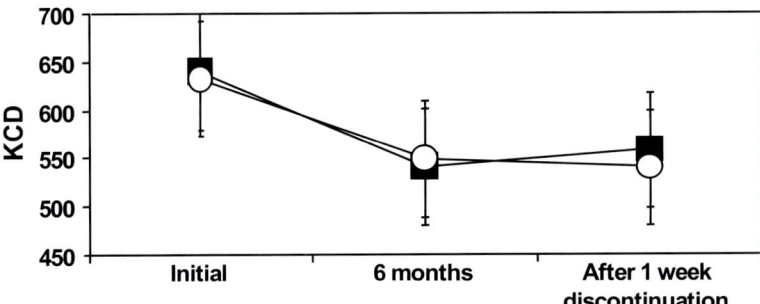

Figure 3.37 Posterior stromal keratocyte density (cells/mm^2) before lens wear (initial), after six months of wear, and one week after discontinuing lens wear in eyes wearing a PureVision lens (white circles) and an Acuvue 2 lens (black squares). Error bars represent ±1 standard deviation

(1997). This decrease did not seem to be dependent on the oxygen performance of the lens, suggesting that hypoxia is not an aetiological factor. Furthermore, these results could not be explained by the presence of oedema because the decrease in posterior stromal KCD noted at six months was still evident one week after ceasing lens wear, at which time the residual oedema had resolved.

It may be that keratocyte loss is related to some mechanical effect. For example, it has been reported that other mechanical effects, such as debridement of the epithelium, are also associated with cell loss (Campos *et al.*, 1994). As a further comparison, there is a reduction in posterior stromal cell density soon after photorefractive keratectomy of about 6% compared with the 14% decrease found in this work (Erie *et al.*, 1999). Wilson *et al.* (1996) detected cell shrinkage, blebbing with formation of membrane-bound bodies, condensation and fragmentation of the chromatin, and DNA fragmentation in anterior stromal keratocytes after the epithelium was damaged by creating scrape wounds. The authors concluded that the disappearance of keratocytes from the underlying anterior stroma following epithelial debridement is mediated by apoptosis. However, the contact lens-induced reduction in KCD reported by Morgan *et al.* (2000) only occurred in the posterior stroma. Certainly, further studies are required to more fully document lens-induced stromal KCD reduction, to shed light on the aetiology of this phenomenon, and to determine if there are any clinical ramifications.

Stromal microdots

Various authors have noted apparently benign, deep stromal opacities in the corneas of contact lens wearers. Pimenides *et al.* (1996) reported four such cases, in which the opacities appeared to be either white, grey or brown; they could be distinguished from infiltrates (which typically reside in the anterior half of the stroma) because these opacities were located deep in the stroma. Similar posterior stromal opacities were reported by Brooks *et al.* (1986), Gobbels *et al.* (1989), Remeijer *et al.* (1990) and Holland *et al.* (1995). Some of these authors attributed their observations to the effects of chronic hypoxia and linked the appearance to endothelial dysfunction.

In 1997, Böhnke and Masters published an alarming report of the confocal microscopic appearance of highly reflective 'microdot deposits' throughout the corneal stroma. These microdots, which could be the magnified appearance of deep stromal opacities, are seen with the confocal microscope as small discrete brightly reflective spots or dots scattered throughout the stroma; they are generally round or oval in shape, and vary in diameter from about 1 to 4 μm (Figure 3.13). Böhnke and Masters (1997) characterized this observation as being indicative of a disease, and established a grading scale to quantify the severity of this disease process in various groups of lens wearers and non-lens wearers. All 13 patients who had worn soft contact lens for an average of 26 years displayed panstromal microdot deposits with a mean score of 3.1 (range 1–4). In the hard contact lens group (average 25 years wear), 11 of 11 subjects had a mean score of 1.9 (range 1–4) for corneal microdot deposits. In the control group, none of 29 patients had stromal microdot deposits. The authors concluded that stromal microdot degeneration as observed with confocal microscopy may be the early stage of a significant corneal disease, which eventually may affect large numbers of patients after decades of contact lens wear.

Because of the profound implications of the finding of Böhnke and Masters (1997), we conducted an experiment in an attempt to replicate their findings. The cornea of one eye in each of 13 patients (age 32 ± 7 years) who had worn contact lenses for an average of 8.2 years was imaged using the confocal microscope, as was the cornea of one eye in each of 13 age- and sex-matched control subjects who had never worn contact lenses. Considerable variation in the intensity of microdots was observed throughout the stroma of a given eye; therefore, three frames from the confocal video sequence that displayed the greatest number of microdots were selected for analysis. To facilitate quantification of the severity of microdots, a microdot grading scale was constructed, along the lines of that devised by Böhnke and Masters (1997), from a series of five images depicting the span from 'no microdots observed' (Grade 0) to a severe case of microdots (Grade 4) (Figure 3.38).

| Grade 0 | Grade 1 | Grade 2 | Grade 3 | Grade 4 |

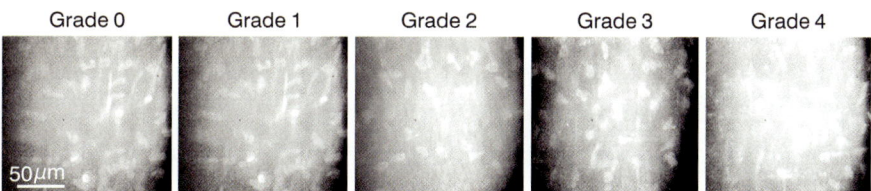

Figure 3.38 Grading scale for assessing the effects of stromal microdots using the confocal microscope

Microdot deposits were observed in the stroma of all 13 lens wearers, with a mean severity of grade 2.0 ± 1.1. In the control group, microdots were observed in 10 of the 13 subjects, with a mean severity in the 10 eyes displaying microdots of 1.5 ± 0.7. The difference in the severity of microdots was statistically significant ($t = -2.47$, $P < 0.02$). The microdots had an identical appearance in lens-wearing and control subjects, apart from the difference in grading. They were all fairly similar in size (1–2 μm diameter).

The fact that microdot deposits are observed in all subjects, whether contact lenses have been worn or not, suggests that this phenomenon cannot be properly characterized as a disease. However, the higher grading assigned to microdots in lens wearers indicates that contact lens wear is exacerbating otherwise normal corneal morphological features. It should also be recognized that it is not possible at present to determine whether the appearance of microdots is related to the contact lenses or the solutions used in conjunction with lens wear. Clearly, this is an issue that requires further investigation.

Endothelial blebs

The first clue that contact lenses could alter the corneal endothelium came from Zantos and Holden (1977), who noted that the endothelial mosaic undergoes a dramatic alteration in appearance within minutes of inserting a contact lens. Specifically, they reported observing a number of black, non-reflecting areas in the endothelial mosaic – which they called blebs – and an apparent increase in the separation between cells. These changes can be observed under high magnification (40×) using the slit lamp (Figure 3.39).

The aetiology of this phenomenon is now well understood. Endothelial blebs are thought to occur as a result of contact lens-induced epithelial acidosis. Two separate factors induce this acidic shift:

1. An increase in carbonic acid due to retardation of carbon dioxide efflux (hypercapnia) by a contact lens.
2. Increased levels of lactic acid as a result of lens-induced oxygen deprivation (hypoxia) and the consequent increase in anaerobic metabolism.

When silicone elastomer contact lenses are worn, such metabolic changes do not take place because of the extremely high oxygen permeability of such lenses (Holden et al., 1985b).

The nature of cellular changes occurring in the endothelium that give rise to blebs has been inferred from histological examination of ex vivo corneas and simple optical models. Histological studies of the endothelial bleb response were conducted by Vannas et al. (1984) using (1) corneas from eyes that were enucleated (because of melanomas) and (2) corneas of beating-heart, brain-death cadavers. The 'blebbed' endothelium displayed oedema of the nuclear area of cells, intracellular fluid vacuoles and fluid spaces between cells. Thus, endothelial blebs appear to be the result of a local oedema phenomenon, whereby the posterior surface of the 'blebbed' endothelial cell is bulged towards the aqueous. The endothelial cell bulges in the posterior direction because this represents the path of least resistance; i.e. the posterior stromal surface (in the region of the posterior limiting lamina) provides much greater resistance to endothelial cell swelling than the aqueous humour. Confocal microscopy may be able to provide further insights into this mechanism.

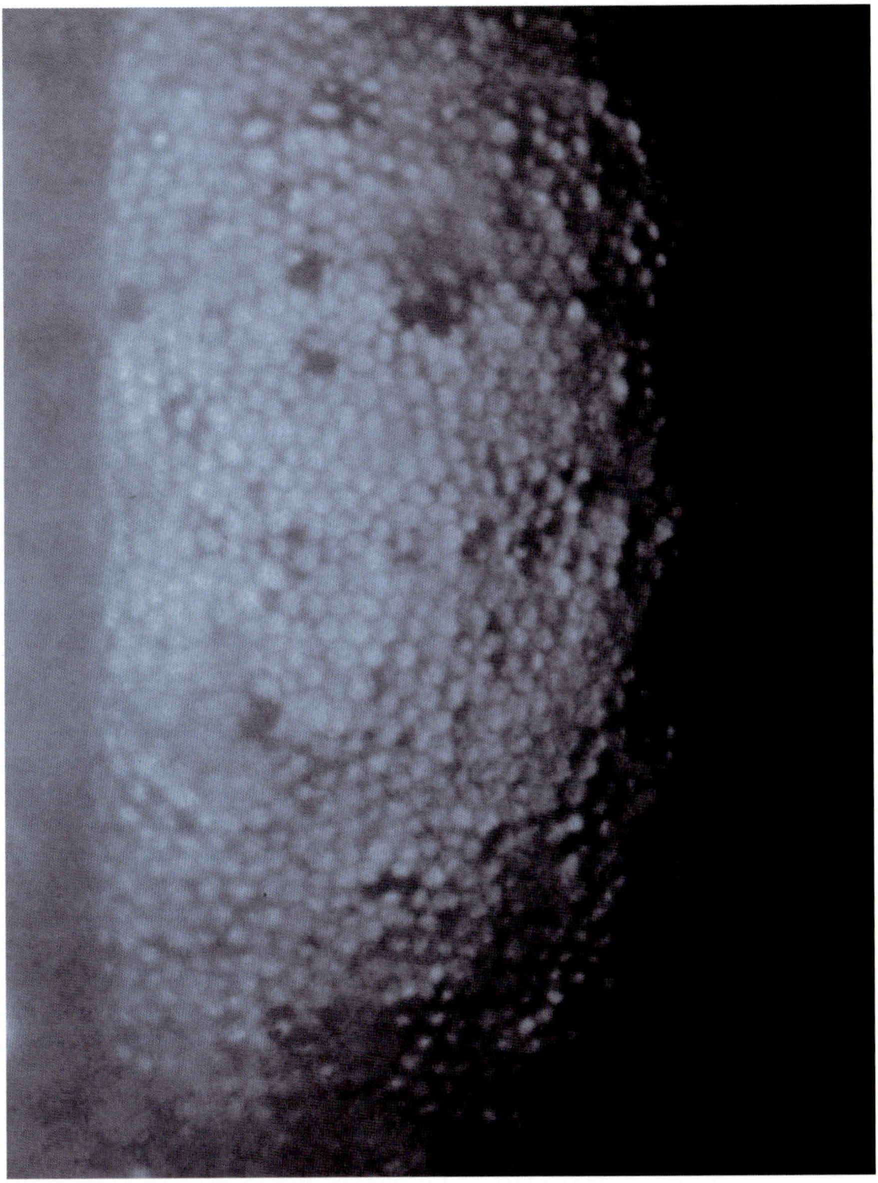

Figure 3.39 Endothelial blebs seen here as apparent black holes using the slit lamp. (Courtesy of Steve Zantos)

Efron (1999) constructed a simple optical model to explain the appearance of blebs (Figure 3.40). When the endothelium is viewed using specular reflection, light rays reflect from the tissue plane corresponding to the interface between the posterior surface of the endothelium and the aqueous humour. This interface acts as the reflective surface because it represents a significant change in tissue refractive index. The light rays that are reflected from this interface give rise to an observed image of an essentially flat (or slightly undulating) and otherwise featureless endothelial cell mosaic. Light rays which strike 'blebbed' endothelial cells are deflected away from the observa-

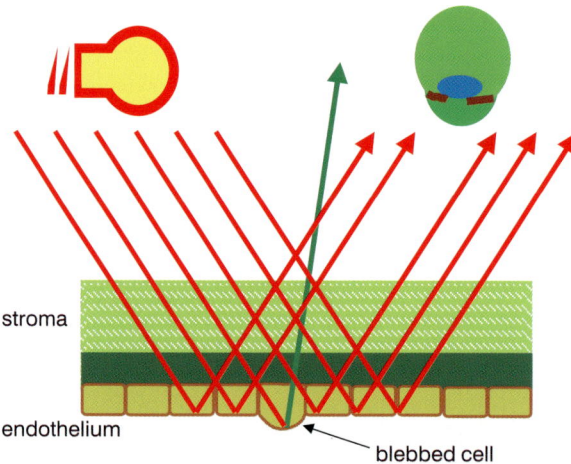

stroma

endothelium

blebbed cell

Figure 3.40 Optical model of the appearance of endothelial blebs with a slit lamp. The red light rays reflect off the posterior endothelium–aqueous interface, allowing that surface to be viewed in specular reflection. The green light ray is deflected away from the eye of the observer by the blebbed cell, giving the illusion of a black hole

tion path, leaving a corresponding small area of darkness. Thus, an endothelial bleb is simply an individual endothelial cell (or group of adjacent cells) that has become swollen and bulged in the direction of the aqueous humour, giving rise to the compelling optical illusion that the cell (or cells) has disappeared.

A study was conducted to observe the bleb response with a confocal microscope. Images were obtained from each eye of 15 normal subjects (age range 19–36 years; mean 26 ± 6 years) before and after 20 minutes wear of a $+5.50\,\mathrm{D}$ 58% water content hydrogel lens in one eye. The extent of the bleb response was graded using Efron Grading Scales (Efron, 1999) (see Figure 1.13 on page 17); the images were also assessed qualitatively.

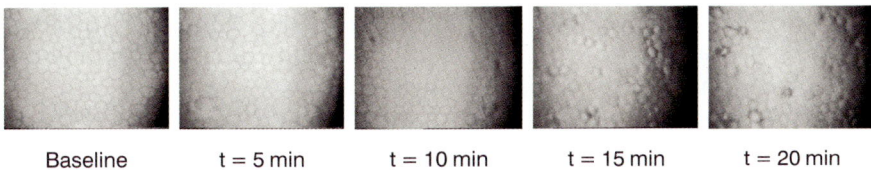

| Baseline | t = 5 min | t = 10 min | t = 15 min | t = 20 min |

Figure 3.41 Confocal microscope images of the development of endothelial blebs over a 20-minute time period

After 20 minutes of lens wear, the mean bleb response in the lens-wearing eye was 1.0 (range 0.0–3.2). Two subjects did not display blebs. No blebs were observed in the non-lens-wearing eyes. Individual blebbed cells, comprising a bright central spot surrounded by a darker annulus, were observed in the endothelium of most subjects.

In one subject, the endothelium was imaged at baseline and over a time sequence of 5, 10, 15 and 20 minutes of lens wear (Figure 3.41). The time sequence reveals the initial appearance of a dark border, which broadens into a thick dark annulus after 15 to 20 minutes of lens wear (Figure 3.42). An optical model is used to illustrate the different

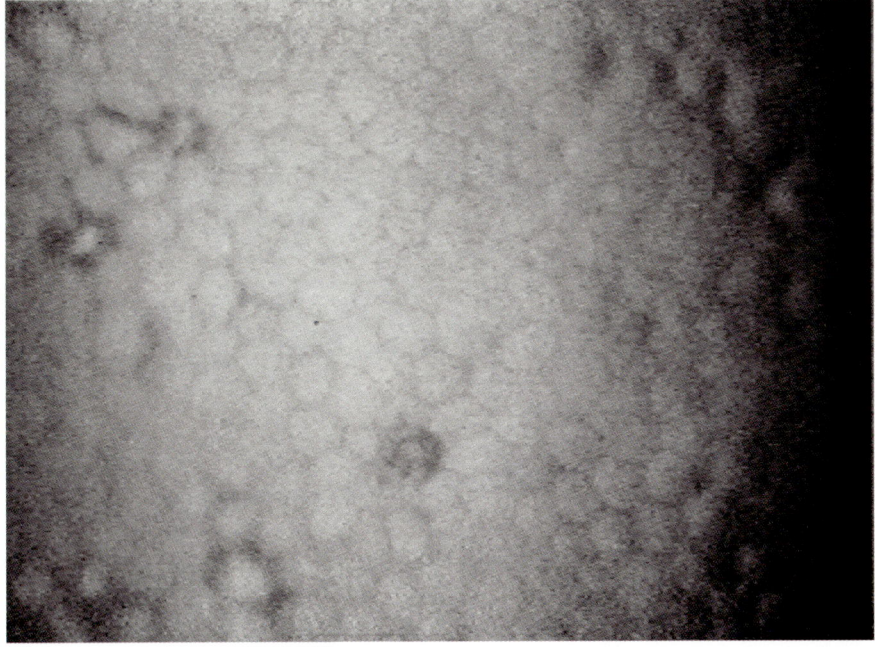

Figure 3.42 Enlargement of a confocal microscope image of bleb formations, showing a bright centre surrounded by a thick dark annulus. The surrounding unaffected endothelium reflects brightly

appearance of endothelial blebs using confocal microscopy (Figure 3.43) versus that seen with the slit lamp (see Figure 3.40). This model employs normal light reflection because light rays pass to and from the endothelium through the confocal microscope objective lens via a normal pathway. This is different from specular microscopy on the slit lamp, whereby angular light reflection is employed to observe the endothelium (Figure 3.40). It can be seen from the confocal model that

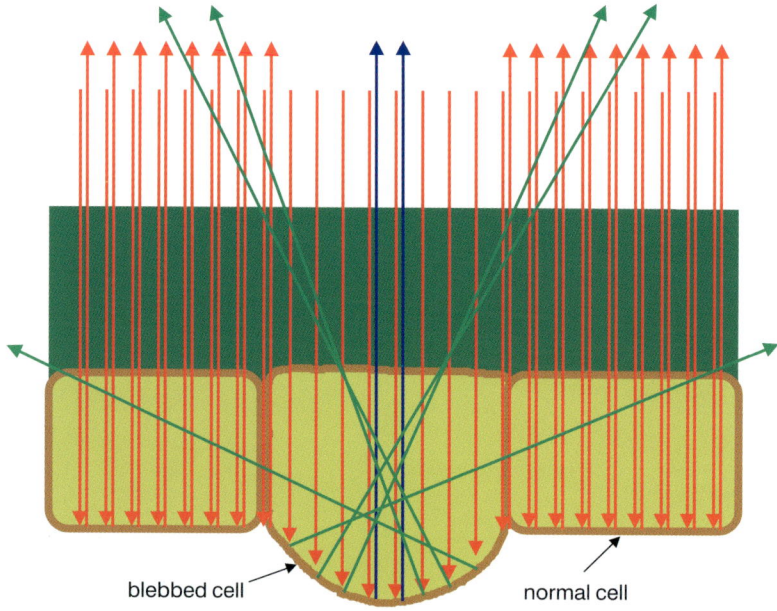

blebbed cell   normal cell

Figure 3.43 Optical model of the appearance of endothelial blebs with a confocal microscope. The red light rays reflect off the posterior endothelium–aqueous interface, allowing that surface to be viewed in specular reflection. The green light rays are deflected away from the eye of the observer by the sloping sides of the blebbed cell, giving rise to the appearance of a dark annulus. The blue rays are reflected normally from the apical region of the blebbed cell, resulting in the centre of the blebbed cell appearing bright

light is normally reflected from the 'non-blebbed' endothelium and the apex of the blebbed endothelial cell, all of which will appear bright. The sloping sides of the blebbed cell reflect light away from the objective and thus appear dark. This model therefore explains the confocal appearance of a blebbed cell as having a dark annulus surrounding a bright central spot. These observations are consistent with the prevailing theory that blebs represent swelling of individual endothelial cells in the posterior direction.

Acanthamoeba keratitis

Acanthamoeba can cause a severe, devastating keratitis that often eludes diagnosis and is resistant to treatment. Acanthamoebas are ubiquitous unicellular free-living parasites that are found in water (swimming pools, hot tubs, tap water, contact lens solutions), air and soil. The life cycle consists of two stages; the active trophozoite and the dormant cyst.

Acanthamoeba cysts are about 9–27 µm in diameter with a wrinkled exocyst and polyhedral endocyst (Nagington *et al.*, 1974). In cystic form, acanthamoeba is highly resistant to the immune response of the host and to harsh environments, including temperature extremes, changes in pH, standard chlorination of water, and many antimicrobial agents (Winchester *et al.*, 1995).

The trophozoite, measuring 15–45 µm in diameter, is mobile and tracks in wavy lines when plated on agar. It derives its nutrition from bacteria, yeast and other unicellular organisms. When exposed to unfavourable environmental conditions, the trophozoite encysts, forming a double wall comprising a thicker outer wall and thinner inner wall (Winchester *et al.*, 1995).

Risk factors for keratitis include contact lens wear, corneal trauma and exposure to contaminated water. Any of these phenomena can cause keratitis that is extremely painful, often resistant to treatment, and commonly requires penetrating keratoplasty.

The best hope for successful treatment is early diagnosis. Early signs of *Acanthamoeba* keratitis tend to be rather non-specific, and this condition is frequently misdiagnosed as herpes simplex or *Pseudomonas* keratitis (see Chapter 2). Furthermore, current methods of diagnosis are unreliable and usually have a fairly high rate of false negatives. Present diagnostic methods include corneal culture and stromal biopsy. Because these methods are invasive, they are often postponed until there is a high index of suspicion for the disease and when there has been no response to treatments for bacteria, viral and/or fungal keratitis (Winchester *et al.*, 1995).

Earlier confocal microscopic observations on rabbits and *in vitro* tissue samples were quickly followed by direct *in vivo* observations of human patients. Various authors have demonstrated the utility of confocal microscopy in the detection of *Acanthamoeba* keratitis (Cavanagh *et al.*, 1993; Auran *et al.*, 1994; Winchester *et al.*, 1995; Pfister *et al.*, 1996; Mathers *et al.*, 2000). Earlier work with confocal microscopes using pinhole disc technology was fraught with difficulty as a result of the aversion patients displayed to the very high illumination required. The more recently introduced slit scanning confocal microscope has proved to be much more patient-friendly, because of the lower light levels required to obtain a good image, and the less invasive non-contact distance-immersion objective. In our laboratory, confocal microscopy is well tolerated by patients (who may otherwise be in a great deal of pain). Patients experience no discomfort or adverse effects in the course of imaging the cornea, and there is no evidence of significant ocular trauma following the procedure. Nevertheless, a high degree of patient cooperation and steady fixation is required for successful imaging, and the procedure may be difficult to perform on children or highly debilitated patients.

Here is a case report from our laboratory (O'Donnell and Efron, 1999). A 70-year-old woman who had recently returned from a beach holiday presented with a unilateral red eye, severe ocular pain, blurred vision and photophobia (Figure 3.44). The patient, who was a long-term daily soft

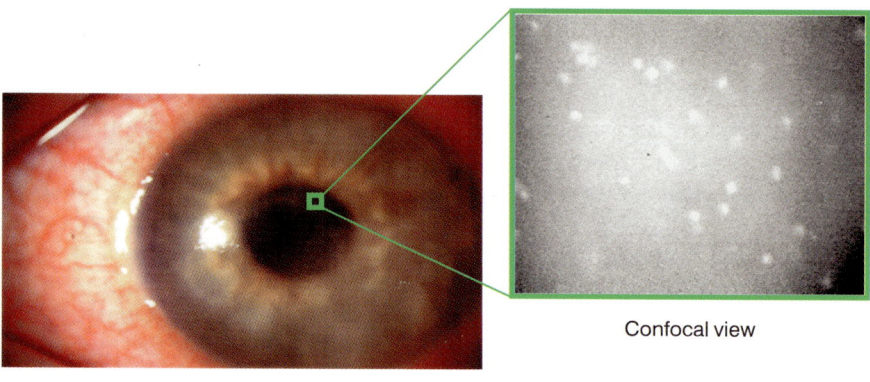

Confocal view

Slit lamp view

Figure 3.44 Slit lamp appearance (left) and confocal microscope image (right; courtesy of Maldonado-Codina and O'Donnell, 1999) of the cornea of a patient suffering from *Acanthamoeba* keratitis

contact lens wearer, had noticed that her right eye was red and sore after swimming while wearing her lenses. She was examined by an ophthalmologist and was suspected to have an *Acanthamoeba* infection. To confirm the diagnosis she was referred to the Department of Optometry and Neuroscience at UMIST to have her eye observed using a confocal microscope.

Confocal microscopy of the anterior segment of the right eye revealed the presence of highly reflective white spherical opacities varying in size from 5 to 18 μm in diameter (Figure 3.44, inset). The opacities were randomly distributed throughout the full depth of the stroma. No keratocytes could be observed anywhere in the stroma. In the mid-stroma, faint images of stromal nerves could sometimes be detected. The endothelial cells could not be imaged. The reason for the failure to observe stromal keratocytes and endothelial cells is unclear but may be related to the presumed high levels of oedema present. These observations confirmed the diagnosis of *Acanthamoeba* keratitis in this patient. The appearance of the cysts is entirely consistent with that described in previous reports, in terms of distribution, size, shape and light reflection characteristics. *Acanthamoeba* cysts can be differentiated from microdots because the former are large (5–18 µm in diameter) and more intensely distributed, and the latter are small (1–4 µm in diameter) and are seen in the presence of stromal keratocytes.

Acanthamoeba cannot be reliably diagnosed from clinical findings alone and successful medical treatment depends on initiating therapy early in the disease process. The confocal microscope provides a significant advantage in diagnosing and managing *Acanthamoeba* keratitis due to its ability to image the parasite in the cornea *in vivo* during the early stages of the infection. It is able to image the *Acanthamoeba* cysts because of the enhanced lateral resolution of the confocal microscope (1 µm) versus the more limited resolution of the slit lamp (20–30 µm). In addition, the high-contrast 'optical sections' that comprise the confocal microscopic images obviate the need for staining, and the capacity to image the cornea in real time offers the distinct advantage of facilitating an immediate clinical diagnosis.

Confocal microscopy is an inexpensive test to perform clinically once the cost of the instrument has been recovered. It also offers the potential for long-term savings by early diagnosis and therefore earlier treatment and subsequent avoidance of penetrating keratoplasty procedures. Because this test is non-invasive, it can be performed even when there is a fairly low index of suspicion for this disease. Besides enabling one to make the initial diagnosis and monitor the response to treatment, it also can be used to check for recurrence after treatment has been discontinued or following penetrating keratoplasty.

In conclusion, the confocal microscope has quickly emerged as a fast, safe and sensitive diagnostic tool for the detection and diagnosis of *Acanthamoeba*, characterizing its precise morphological form (trophozoite versus cyst), grading the severity of the condition, monitoring the progression of the disease, and evaluating the efficacy of various treatment modalities.

Conclusions

The development of the slit-scanning confocal microscope has heralded the introduction of a whole new era in ocular science and medicine. It is now possible to view structures of the cornea at a cellular level, and consequently phenomena that have previously only been imaged at low magnification and resolution can now be reinvestigated to develop a better understanding of normal corneal structure and function and abnormal corneal conditions. The implications of this technology for generating a better understanding of corneal disease are profound, and detailed research is at an early stage. The potential for developing a greater appreciation of contact lens-related ocular reactions is also immense, and this chapter has provided an overview of some preliminary observations in this regard.

The only factor preventing widespread deployment and use of this instrument at present is the high cost, which is understandable when one considers the significant financial investments that have fuelled the initial research and development of this very complex technology. At this point in time, therefore, the confocal microscope is available primarily in research clinics and hospital departments. There is no doubt that the cost of confocal microscopes will drop significantly in the coming years as the real clinical worth of this technology becomes more widely appreciated and demand begins to grow.

Some clinicians may be wondering whether the introduction of the confocal microscope will mean the demise of the slit lamp, which has served the ophthalmic professions well for over a century in the investigation of anterior eye disease. However, the drawing of such a conclusion would indicate a misunderstanding of the real worth of the confocal microscope in a clinical setting. The slit lamp, with its full colour, wide-field view, low-to-medium magnification, binocular objective and highly versatile illumination system, will always remain the instrument of first choice in examining any ocular disease or contact lens-related disorder of the anterior eye. It is essential to be able to view the whole of the affected tissue (e.g. the cornea), rather than just the microscopic region of interest, as well as adjacent unaffected regions of the same tissue. It is also critical to be able to view other nearby ocular structures (the limbus, conjunctiva, eyelids, etc.) for the presence or absence of concurrent pathology, so that an overall initial diagnosis can be made. Following a mandatory initial examination with the slit lamp, the confocal microscope can be employed to image specific regions of interest in the cornea more closely in order to define more precisely the tissue pathology.

The ideal consulting room of an eye care practitioner would house a slit lamp and a confocal microscope side by side. Practitioners who have access to a confocal microscope will marvel at the ability to be able to view the cornea at a cellular level. Certainly, patients will benefit from the greater overall diagnostic synergy conferred by the combined application of the slit lamp and confocal microscope.

References

Auran, J. D., Starr, M. B., Koester, C. J. and Labombardi, V. J. (1994) In-vivo scanning slit confocal microscopy of acanthamoeba-keratitis – a case-report. *Cornea*, **13**, 183–185.

Bansal, A. K., Mustonen, R. K. and McDonald, M. B. (1997) High resolution in vivo scanning confocal microscopy of the cornea in long term contact lens wear. *Invest. Ophthalmol. Vis. Sci.*, **38**, S138.

Böhnke, M. and Masters, B. R. (1997) Long term contact lens wear induces a corneal degeneration with microdot deposits in the corneal stroma. *Ophthalmology*, **104**, 1887–1896.

Böhnke, M. and Masters, B. R. (1999) Confocal microscopy of the cornea. *Prog. Ret. Eye. Res.*, **18**, 553–682.

Bourne, W. M., Nelson, L. R. and Hodge, D. O. (1996) Morphologic changes in human corneal endothelium over a ten-year period. *Invest. Ophthalmol. Vis. Sci.*, **37**, S702.

Bron, A. J., Tripathi, R. C. and Tripathi, B. J. (1997) *Wolff's Anatomy of the Eye and Orbit*. Chapman & Hall Medical.

Brooks, A. M. V., Westmore, R., Grant, G. and Robertson, I. F. (1986) Deep corneal stromal opacities with contact lenses. *Aust. New Zeal. J. Ophthalmol.*, **14**, 243–249.

Campos, M., Raman, S., Lee, M. and McDonald, P. J. (1994) Keratocyte loss after different methods of de-epithelialization. *Ophthalmology*, **101**, 890–894.

Cavanagh, H. D, Petroll, W. M., Alizadeh, H. *et al.* (1993) Clinical and diagnostic use of in-vivo confocal microscopy in patients with corneal disease. *Ophthalmology*, **100**, 1444–1454.

Efron, N. (1999) *Contact Lens Complications*. Butterworth-Heinemann/Optician.

Efron, N., Mutalib, H. A., Hiang, K. H. and Perez-Gomez, I. (1999) Confocal microscopy of the edematous cornea following overnight lens wear. *Optom. Vis. Sci.*, **76**, S17.

Erie, J. C., Patel, S. V., McLaren, J. W. *et al.* (1999) Keratocyte density in vivo after photorefractive keratectomy in humans. *Trans. Am. Ophthalmol. Soc.*, **97**, 221–236

Gobbels, M., Wahning, A. and Spitznas, M. (1989) Endothelial function in contact lens-induced deep corneal opacities. *Fortschr. Ophthalmol.*, **86**, 448–450.

Hahnel, C., Somodi, S., Weiss, D. G. and Guthoff, R. F. (2000) The keratocyte network of human cornea: A three-dimensional study using confocal laser scanning fluorescence microscope. *Cornea*, **19**, 185–193.

Holden, B. A., Mertz, G. W. and McNally, J. J. (1983) Corneal swelling response to contact lenses worn under extended wear conditions. *Invest. Ophthalmol. Vis. Sci.*, **24**, 218–226.

Holden, B. A., Sweeney, D. F., Vannas, A. *et al.* (1985a) Effects of long-term extended contact lens wear on the human cornea. *Invest. Ophthalmol. Vis. Sci.* **26**, 1489–1501.

Holden, B. A, Williams, L. and Zantos, S. G. (1985b) The etiology of transient endothelial changes in the human cornea. *Invest. Ophthalmol. Vis. Sci.*, **26**, 1354–1359.

Holland, E. J., Lee, R. M., Bucci, F. A. *et al.* (1995) Mottled cyan opacification of the posterior cornea in contact lens wearers. *Am. J. Ophthalmol.*, **119**, 620–626.

Jalbert, I. and Stapleton, F. (1999) Effect of lens wear on corneal stroma: preliminary findings. *Aust. New Zeal. J. Ophthalmol.*, **27**, 211–213.

Jalbert, I., Stapleton, F., Papas, E. *et al.* (2000) Surface epithelial cell size measured in vivo using confocal microscopy in an underestimate of size measured with contact lens cytology. *Invest. Ophthalmol. Vis. Sci.*, **41**, S913.

Kiely, P. M., Carney, L. G. and Smith, G. (1982) Diurnal variations of corneal topography and thickness. *Am. J. Optom. Physiol. Opt.*, **59**, 976–982.

LaHood, D. and Grant, T. (1990) Striae and folds as indicators of corneal oedema. *Optom. Vis. Sci.*, **67**, S196.

LaHood, D., Sweeney, D. F. and Holden, B. A. (1988) Overnight corneal edema with hydrogel, rigid gas-permeable and silicone-elastomer contact lenses. *Int. Contact Lens Clin.*, **15**, 149–152.

Lemp, M. A. and Mathers, W. D. (1989) Corneal epithelial cell movement in humans. *Eye*, **3**, 438–445.

Lemp, M. A., Dilly, P. N. and Boyde, A. (1986) Tandem-scanning (confocal) microscopy of the full-thickness cornea. *Cornea*, **4**, 205–209.

Liu, Z. G. and Pflugfelder, S. C. (2000) The effects of long-term contact lens wear on corneal thickness, curvature, and surface regularity. *Ophthalmology*, **107**, 105–111.

Maldonado-Codina, C. and O'Donnell, C. (1999) A new paradigm: in vivo confocal microscopy. *Optician*, **217** (5705), 18–19; **217** (5706), 14–16.

Malik, N. S., Moss, S. J., Ahmed, N. *et al.* (1992) Ageing of the human corneal stroma: structural and biochemical changes. *Biochem. Biophys. Acta*, **1138**, 222–228.

Masters, B. R. and Farmer, M. A. (1993) Three-dimensional confocal microscopy and visualization of the *in situ* cornea. *Comp. Med. Imag. Graph.*, **17**, 211–219.

Masters, B. R. and Thaer, A. A. (1994) Real-time scanning slit confocal microscopy of the *in vivo* human cornea. *Appl. Optics*, **33**, 695–701.

Mathers, W. D., Nelson, S. E., Lane, J. L. *et al.* (2000) Confirmation of confocal microscopy diagnosis of *Acanthamoeba* keratitis using polymerase chain reaction analysis. *Arch. Ophthalmol.*, **118**, 178–183.

Minsky, M. (1988) Memoir on inventing the confocal scanning microscope. *Scanning*, **10**, 128–138.

Moller-Pedersen, T. (1997) A comparative study of human corneal keratocyte and endothelial cell density during aging. *Cornea*, **19**, 333–338.

Morgan, P. B., Gomez-Perez, I. and Efron, N. (2000) A comparative assessment of continuous wear lenses. Paper presented to the 19th European Symposium on Contact Lenses, Berlin, Germany, 15 October 2000.

Mustonen, R. K., McDonald, M. B., Srivannaboon, S. *et al.* (1998) Normal human corneal cell populations evaluated by in vivo scanning slit confocal microscopy. *Cornea*, **17**, 485–492.

Mutalib, H. A. and Efron, N. (1999) Grading scales for corneal edema viewed with a confocal microscope. *Optom. Vis. Sci.*, **76**, S234.

Mutalib, H. A., Perez-Gomez, I., Hollingsworth, J. and Efron, N. (1999) Corneal keratocyte and endothelial cell density in a normal population. *Optom. Vis. Sci.*, **76**, S242.

Nagington, J., Watson, P. G., Playfair, T. J. *et al.* (1974) Amoebic infection of the eye. *Lancet*, **2**, 1537.

O'Donnell, C. and Efron, N. (1999) Confocal microscopy of the cornea after acanthamoeba keratitis. *Optom. Vis. Sci.*, **76**, S50.

O'Leary, D. J., Madgewick, R., Walface, J. and Ang, J. (1998) Size and number of epithelial cells washed from the cornea after contact lens wear. *Optom. Vis. Sci.*, **75**, 692–696.

Oliveira-Soto, L. (1999) Morphology of corneal nerves in soft contact lens wear. A comparative study using confocal microscopy. MSc thesis, University of Manchester Institute of Science and Technology.

Olsen, T. and Ehlers, N. (1984) The thickness of the human cornea as determined by a specular method. *Acta Ophthalmol.*, (Copenh.), **62**, 859–871.

Perez-Gomez, I., Hollingsworth, J., Morgan, P. B. and Efron, N. (2000) A reference grid of the normal human cornea viewed with a confocal microscope. *Optom. Vis. Sci.*, **77**, S153.

Petran, M., Hadravsky, M., Egger, M. D. and Galambos, R. (1968) Tandem-scanning reflected-light microscopy. *J. Opt. Soc. Am.*, **58**, 661–664.

Pfister, D. R., Cameron, J. D., Krachmer, J. H. and Holland, E. J. (1996) Confocal microscopy findings of Acanthamoeba keratitis. *Am. J. Ophthalmol.*, **121**, 119–128.

Pimenides, P., Steele, C. F., McGhee, C. N. J. and Bryce, I. G. (1996) Deep corneal stromal opacities associated with long term contact lens wear. *Br. J. Ophthalmol.*, **80**, 21–24.

Remeijer, L., Van Rij, G., Beekhuis, W. H. *et al.* (1990) Deep corneal stromal opacities in long-term contact lens wear. *Ophthalmology*, **97**, 281–285.

Sarver, M. D. (1971) Striate corneal lines among patients wearing hydrophilic contact lenses. *Am. J. Optom. Physiol. Opt.*, **48**, 762–765.

Tomii, S. and Kinoshita, S. (1994) Observations of human corneal epithelium by tandem scanning confocal microscope. *Scanning*, **16**, 305–306.

Tsubota, K. and Yamada, M. (1992) Corneal epithelial alterations induced by disposable contact-lens wear. *Ophthalmology*, **99**, 1193–1196.

Vannas, A., Holden, B.A., Makitie, J. (1984) The ultrastructure of contact lens induced changes in the human corneal endothelium. *Acta Ophthalmol.*, **62**, 320–333.

Wilson, G. (2000) The epithelium in extended wear. In *Silicone Hydrogels: The Rebirth of Continuous Wear Contact Lenses* (D. F. Sweeney, ed.), pp. 22–44, Butterworth-Heinemann.

Wilson, S. E., He, Y. G., Weng, J. *et al.* (1996) Epithelial injury induces keratocyte apoptosis: Hypothesized role for the interleukin–1 system in the modulation of corneal tissue organization and wound healing. *Exp. Eye Res.*, **62**, 325–337.

Winchester, K., Mathers, W. D., Sutphin, J. E. and Daley, T. E. (1995) Diagnosis of acanthamoeba keratitis in vivo with confocal microscopy. *Cornea*, **14**, 10–17.

Zantos, S. G. and Holden, B. A. (1977) Transient endothelial changes soon after wearing soft contact lenses. *Am. J. Optom. Physiol. Opt.*, **54**, 856–858.

4 Light and electron microscopy

Jan P. G. Bergmanson

Introduction

The gaining of insights into corneal anatomy evaded mankind for a long time. Part of the reason for this ignorance must have been the fact that the cornea is transparent. Therefore, there was not much to see – until something went wrong and transparency was lost (bringing with it a consequent loss of vision). Paradoxically, the slit lamp is of limited assistance when examining a clear cornea, but when transparency is disturbed, focusing on a detail is more easily accomplished.

It was with the advent of the light microscope and the pioneering histologists such as Antony van Leeuwenhoek (1632–1723) of Holland, Sir William Bowman (1816–1892) of Great Britain, and Hans Virchow (1852–1940) of Germany that ocular scientists and clinicians began to learn corneal anatomy (Duke Elder and Wybar, 1961; Albert and Edwards, 1996). With the physical limitations of the light microscope, the learning curve relating to ocular anatomy plateaued early in the twentieth century, and it was only with the advent of the electron microscope that giant leaps forward in knowledge about the cornea have been possible. Pioneers in the field of ocular ultrastructure, to mention a select few, include John Dowling of the USA, Toichiro Kuwabara of Japan, Gordon Ruskell of the UK, Fritiof Sjöstrand of Sweden, George Smelser of the USA, and Brenda and Ramesh Tripathi of the UK and later the USA. Of course, there are many more outstanding anatomists who may be added to this list if space allowed. Today, in the twenty-first century, new technologies bringing great benefits have emerged, such as confocal microscopy and molecular biology, but it should be recognized that there is still no new technology that provides higher resolution than the electron microscope. This chapter, while not exhaustive, attempts to communicate a review of the current state of understanding of the anatomy of the normal and contact lens-wearing cornea, as seen through the light and electron microscopes. An emphasis will be placed upon aspects of particular interest and relevance to contact lens practitioners.

A brief history of light and electron microscopy

In the late nineteenth century, Ernst Abbe shocked his contemporaries by suggesting that the light microscope had reached its limit, justifying this viewpoint on the dependence of the long wavelengths of visible light. Thus, the real limit of the resolution of the light microscope was the light source and not the optics of the lens used (Hayat, 1973). Abbe realized that instruments utilizing shorter wavelengths would be the solution to overcome the limitations of the light microscope. However, it was not until 1932 that the first electron microscope (EM) was developed by Max Knoll and Ernst Ruska in Germany. Metropolitan Vickers, in 1937, was probably the first company to construct a prototype for an electron microscope, while the Siemens Company in Germany was first to commercialize this technology in 1938–39 (Bozzola and Russell, 1992). The transmission electron microscope (TEM) was a revolutionary new tool that required a new set of auxiliary technologies to be developed before it could reach its full potential. For instance, the knives and microtomes used for light microscopy were unable to provide the thin sections required for the TEM, and as a result, the ultramicrotome, the glass knife and later, the diamond knife became essential instruments in the EM lab. Also, the embedding medium had to be changed from the traditional paraffin to the more sophisticated plastic or epoxy material. This merger of technologies took some time to refine and hone, and it was not until the late 1950s and early 1960s that something resembling quality ultrastructure imaging started to appear in biological sciences journals.

The scanning electron microscope (SEM) appeared on the horizon in the late 1950s. Interestingly, the pioneers in scanning tunnelling electron microscopy, Heinrich Rohrer and Gerd Binnig, received the 1986 Nobel Prize for Physics, which was shared with Ernst Ruska.

Instruments offering the incredible resolution of 1–2 angstroms (Å) would be useless unless techniques could be developed to preserve tissue in its natural shape and appearance without creating distracting artefacts. Textbooks have been devoted to this chemical challenge faced by the anatomist studying ultrastructure. In this context, the cornea presents a unique problem to researchers who attempt to achieve optimal fixation of this tissue. The problem to overcome is in part due to the fact that the cornea lacks a blood supply; therefore, the only method by which the cornea may be successfully fixed is immersion. Perfusion of fixatives through the vascular system, which is the only viable solution for most other organs, does not yield optimal results on the cornea. The dense and relatively dehydrated collagenous stroma packed between two cellular layers, which also function as fluid barriers, does not make this task easier. Fortunately, protocols that describe the optimal fixation of the cornea are now available (Doughty *et al.*, 1997). A solution of 2% glutaraldehyde in 80 mM buffer, yielding an osmolarity of 330–340 mOsm/l and a pH of 7.4, has been shown to be particularly useful in achieving good corneal cellular preservation and maintenance of a normal corneal shape with minimal shrinkage or distortion of the tissue.

The normal cornea

This section will provide an overview of the gross anatomy and embryonic development of the normal cornea so that descriptions of microscopic corneal anatomy can be put into a proper perspective. This overview will also foster a better appreciation of subsequent descriptions of the growth mechanisms, transitions, attachment mechanics, and structural and functional interrelationships beween the various corneal layers.

Gross structure and function

The cornea is part of the outer coat and it is also continuous with the conjunctiva and ultimately the skin. Its physiology is uniquely adapted to its functions. The cornea is an avascular structure bathed in fluid – tears anteriorly and aqueous posteriorly. It covers one-sixth of the circumference of the eyeball, with sclera providing for the remaining five-sixths.

The cornea describes an oval shape with the larger diameter being horizontal. A summary of key physical and optical properties of the cornea is given in Table 4.1. In the extreme periphery, the cornea is gradually transformed to sclera. This transitional zone is known as limbus. A number of important structural modifications occur in limbus, but with the exception of the epithelium, they are regarded as outside the scope of this chapter.

Traditionally, the cornea is described as a five-layered structure:

1. epithelium (outermost layer);
2. anterior limiting lamina (Bowman's membrane);
3. stroma;
4. posterior limiting lamina (Descemet's membrane);
5. endothelium (innermost layer).

This may seem inconsistent because the endothelial basement membrane is treated as a separate layer, whereas the epithelial basement membrane is not. Figure 4.1 is a light micrograph of the cornea in cross-section.

Table 4.1 Physical measurements of the cornea	
Diameter	11.7 mm (horizontal) × 10.6 mm (vertical)
Central thickness	535 μm
Radius of curvature	Anterior: 7.8 mm Posterior: 6.2–6.8 mm (varying with the source)
Front surface refractive power	48.83 D
Back surface refractive power	−5.88 D
Total corneal refractive power	43.05 D
Refractive index	1.376
Water content	78%
Collagen content	15%
Other proteins content	5%

Sources: Duke-Elder and Wybar, 1961; Bennett and Rabbetts, 1998; Doughty and Zaman, 2000.

The cornea has two primary functions. First, it serves the dual optical functions of maintaining a transparent 'clear window' to the eye to promote the transmission of light, and refracting light to help focus the object being viewed onto the retina. Indeed, the cornea is responsible for two-thirds of the refraction taking place in the eye. Second, the cornea – being a somewhat rigid fibrous structure with a renewable epithelial surface – protects the delicate intraocular structures from trauma.

Embryology

Useful reviews on corneal and ocular embryology exist in the literature (see Marshall and Grindle, 1978; Bron *et al.*, 1997; Cook *et al.*, 1999). After five weeks of gestation the earliest corneal manifestation – a single layer of ectodermal cells – is noted (Marshall and Grindel, 1978; Bron *et al.*, 1997). This layer will become the corneal epithelium, which adopts an

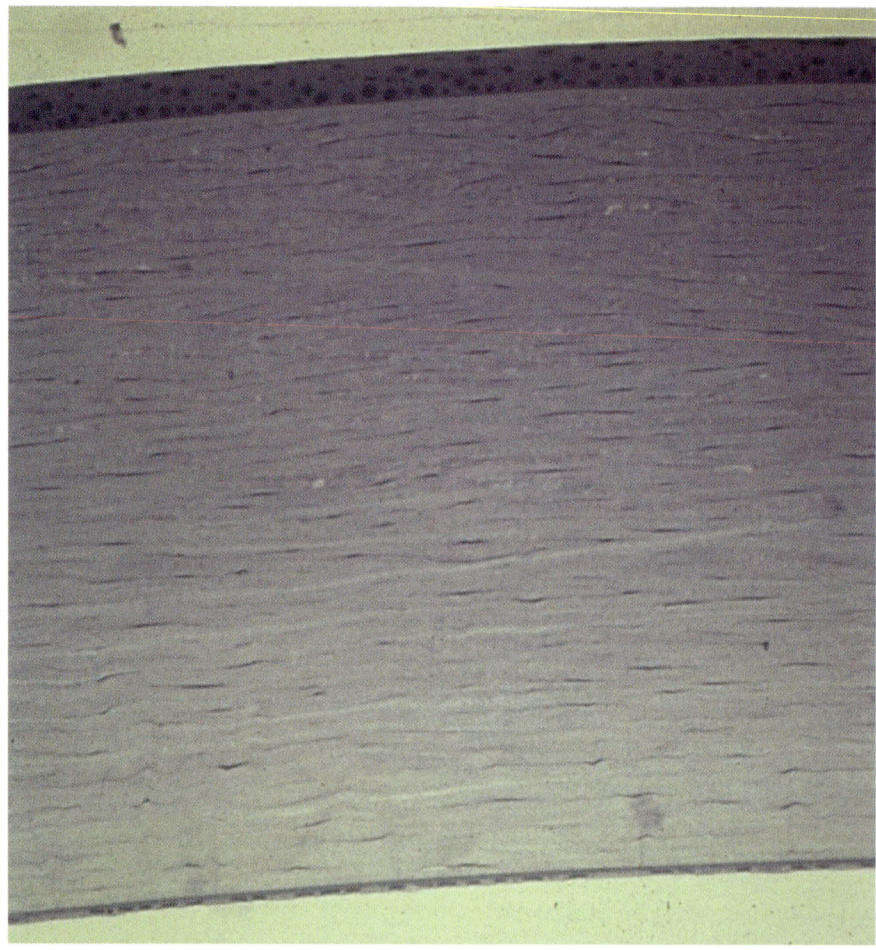

Figure 4.1 Transverse section through the cornea, which is bounded anteriorly by a stratified, non-keratinized epithelium and posteriorly by a single layer of squamous endothelial cells. Stromal tissue occupies the space between these two boundary layers. Within the stroma, dense staining keratocytes, more numerous anteriorly may be noted. Primate. Light micrograph, magnification approximately ×100

almost adult appearance as the fetus opens its eyes after 5–6 months of pregnancy (Bron *et al.*, 1997). At the seven-week interval mesoderm enters to form stromal tissue.

The anterior limiting lamina (Bowman's membrane) appears relatively late in the developing fetus (at 5 months) and appears to be formed by anterior keratocytes that later leave the area to create a cell-free zone (Bron *et al.*, 1997; Cook *et al.*, 1999). The collagenous secretion of stromal cells, later to become keratocytes, produces the corneal lamellae, which increase in number throughout pregnancy (Bron *et al.*, 1997; Cook *et al.*, 1999).

There is some uncertainty regarding the true origin of keratocytes and endothelium. Immunohistochemical work has indicated that both keratocytes and endothelial cells are derived from neural crest cells, which later will differentiate into mesenchymal cells (Hayashi *et al.*, 1986).

Initially the secreted collagen network is loose but gradually the continuous growth creates the denser and more parallel organized collagen bundles termed lamellae. The cornea grows both in thickness, from adding more lamellae, and in width, from elongation of lamellae (Bron *et al.*, 1997; Cook *et al.*, 1999). Adult corneal dimensions are not attained until after birth. For instance, at birth the corneal diameter is about 10 mm, but one year postnatally, corneal diameter has increased to approximately adult proportions at 11.7 mm (Marshall and Grindle, 1978). The adult corneal thickness is 535 μm (Doughty and Zaman, 2000), but the embryological and postnatal timetable to reach this dimension has yet to be determined.

At 40 days of pregnancy, a double row of squamous mesenchymal cells appear posterior to the basal lamina of the two rows of epithelial cells (Cook *et al.*, 1999). This will become the endothelium, which simultaneously will secrete its basement membrane – the posterior limiting lamina (Descemet's membrane). The posterior limiting lamina continues to grow throughout life, while the endothelium will have its adult configuration by birth. Endothelial mitosis ceases at birth.

The earliest signs of ciliary nerves are formed at the eight-week stage at the edge of the optic cup, and during the 12th week, fine neural twigs are present in the stroma (Marshall and Grindle, 1978).

Microscopic anatomy

From a basic science perspective, a comprehensive appreciation of normal tissue morphology makes a critical contribution to understanding how that tissue functions. From a clinical perspective, it is necessary to understand the normal morphology of a tissue, as imaged by a given technique, so that any suspected abnormalities detected with that technique can be identified as such and action taken to remedy the problem. Needless to say, this principle applies to light and electron microscopy. This section provides an overview of the microscopic anatomy of the normal cornea as viewed with these techniques, and serves as a reference against which the contact lens-induced changes described later in this chapter can be appreciated.

Epithelium

The epithelium has a number of anatomical features that can be linked to specific functions. These features include:

- Optical – the epithelium needs to be transparent, and truly the anterior refractive surface of the eye.
- Physical protection – from external trauma. The epithelium constitutes a resilient and renewable protective layer of the ocular surface.
- Fluid barrier – the surface layer of cells contains zonulae occludentes, which prevent an anterior fluid leakage in or out of the cornea.
- Microorganism shield – even in the normal healthy eye there is a flora of microorganisms present in the tear fluids. It is thought that disturbances to the integrity of the ocular surface involve removal or inhibition of this barrier, which may in turn facilitate microbial invasion of the cornea. Only five organisms are known to penetrate the intact epithelium – *Pseudomonas aeruginosa*, *Streptococcus pneumoniae*, *Neisseria gonorrhoeae*, *Haemophilus influenzae*, and *Corynebacterium* spp.
- Tear stabilizer – the microvilli and the microplicae on the epithelial surface are believed to be important in promoting tear stability.

The epithelium is classified as a stratified epithelial layer and it comprises five to seven layers of tightly packed cells. No spaces are evident between the cells. The corneal epithelium shows continuity with the conjunctival epithelium, which itself is continuous with the skin of the eyelid. In the healthy eye, the epithelium is not keratinized. However, in patients with severe dry eye, the epithelium may become keratinized. The absence of keratin in the epithelium explains its fragility when compared to the resilience of the keratinized surface epithelium of skin.

The epithelial layer measures approximately $50.6 \pm 3.9\,\mu m$ in thickness (Li *et al.*, 1997). Three distinct shapes of cells are recognized in the epithelium: 'basal', 'wing' and 'squamous' (or 'superficial') cells. Figures 4.2 and 4.3 show transverse sections through the epithelium as seen with light and electron microscopy, respectively. The basal cells are the most internal and are attached to the basement membrane, which they secrete (Figure 4.4). The wing cells, sometimes called umbrella cells due to their shape, are found immediately external to the single row of basal cells. External to the two or three rows of wing cells are two to three rows of flattened squamous cells. The ocular surface is formed by the most external row of squamous cells. These cells do not represent three different classes of cells, but rather the same cell captured at different stages in life. The life cycle of an epithelial cell has been estimated to be around seven days

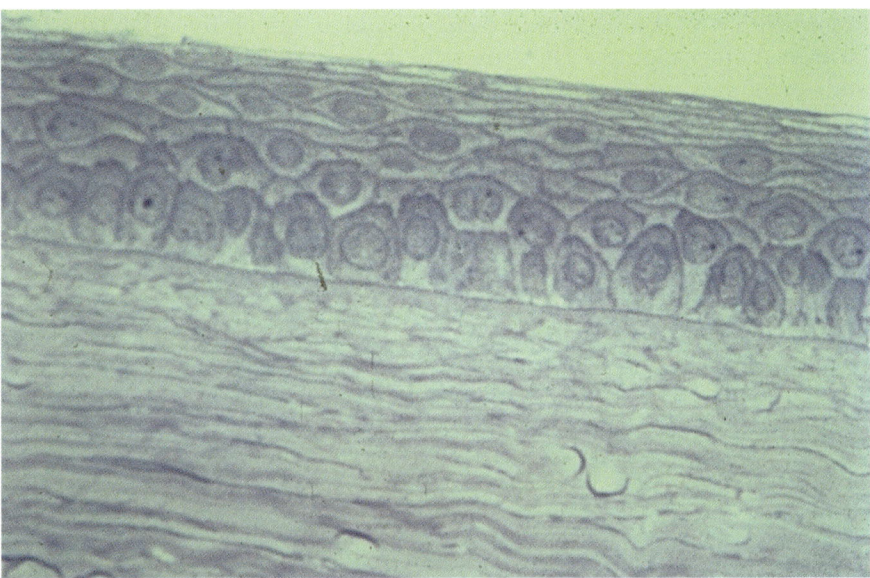

Figure 4.2 Transverse section through the epithelium, which comprises five to seven layers of tightly packed cells. No spaces are present between cells. A basement membrane provides the foundation on which the epithelium is attached to the remainder of the cornea. Primate. Light micrograph, magnification approximately ×250

(Hanna and O'Brien, 1960). The outline of the external squamous cells along the corneal surface forms an irregular pattern and the side exposed to the tears is densely populated by microvilli and microplicae.

Epithelial renewal was previously believed to be accomplished through simple cell division of basal cells across the entire cornea. Following division the cells would move straight towards the corneal surface and desquamate into the tears. However, mounting scientific and clinical evidence suggests a more complex epithelial arrangement for renewal. For instance, destruction of limbal and conjunctival epithelium through trauma or disease leads to loss of epithelial integrity in the central cornea. This realization led to the 'X-Y-Z hypothesis' of Thoft and Friend (1983), which states that the proliferation of basal cells (X) together with a centripetal movement of peripherally located cells (Y) equals the desquamation rate (Z) at the surface (Figure 4.5). The Thoft–Friend hypothesis suggests that to remain healthy the central cornea cannot depend on local mitosis but requires a net flux of cells from the periphery.

The current thinking is that the renewal of the corneal epithelium is the responsibility of stem cells located in the limbal region (Kruse, 1994; Zieske, 1994). These cells appear to be underdeveloped or primitive.

Identification of stem cells is difficult and is generally established by indirect methodologies. They are genetically geared for a long life span and exhibit a very slow turnover life cycle. Stem cells have an unrestricted capability for producing identical daughter cells via mitosis, which is either symmetric or asymmetric. Asymmetric division occurs when one daughter cell stays to provide replenishment to the stem cell pool (Dua and Azuara-Blanco, 2000).

The daughter stem cells produced in the cornea are known as transient amplifying (TA) cells (Cotsarelis *et al.*, 1989) and they will migrate centripetally. During this migration, the TA cells will divide a few times before reaching the surface to desquamate. These cells may occasionally

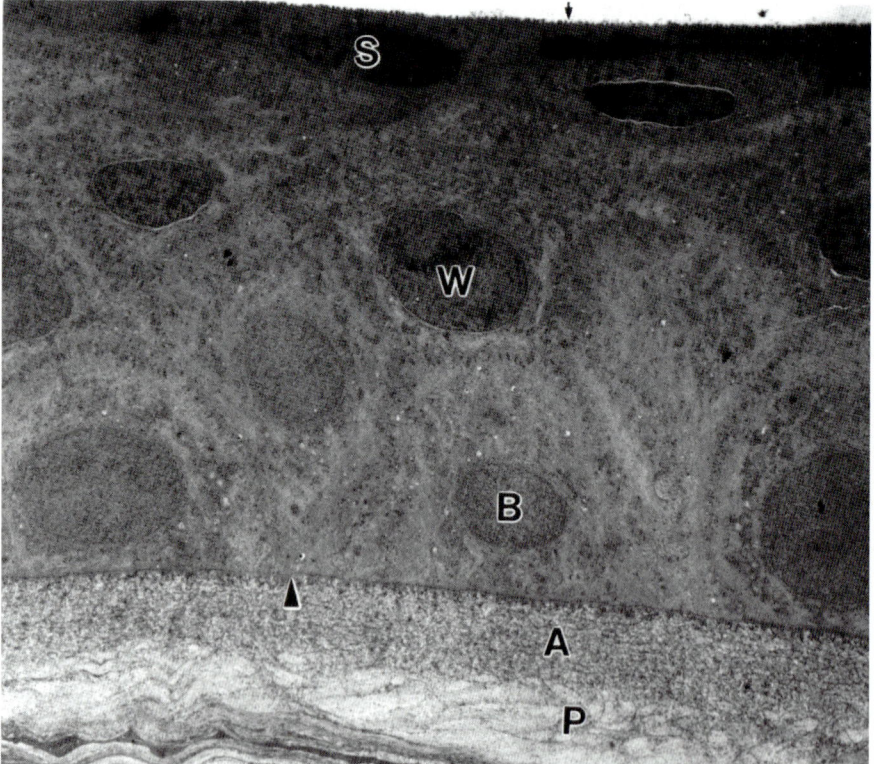

Figure 4.3 Transverse section through epithelium. The epithelial surface is anteriorly lined by microvilli (arrow) and posteriorly by a basement membrane (triangle). The cells forming the epithelium are classified according to their shape and location as basal (B), wing (W), and squamous (S) cells; here the letters 'B', 'W' and 'S' are overlaid on the cell nuclei. Internally, the basement membrane faces the anterior limiting lamina (A), which itself internally merges into the stroma (P). Primate. Electron micrograph, magnification approximately ×5100

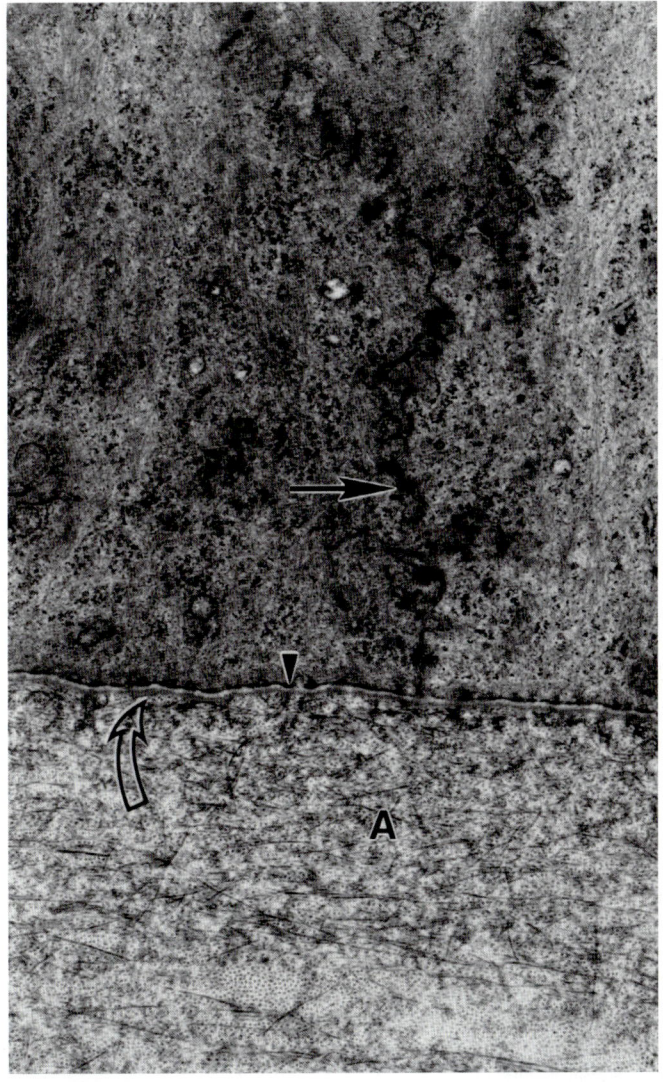

Figure 4.4 Transverse section through basal epithelium. The interdigitated outline of the tightly packed epithelium can be seen; there are no spaces between the cells. Numerous desmosomes (arrow) are found between cells. Hemidesmosomes (triangle), which hold cells to the basement membrane, are dotted along the basal side of the cell. Internally, the anterior limiting lamina (A) lines the basement membrane, with which a series of fine Type VII collagen fibres (open arrow) are linked. Primate. Electron micrograph, magnification ×11 200

divide in the wing cell layers on their way to the corneal surface (Bergmanson, 1981). It follows that the central cornea does not have resident stem cells and that these essential cells are located in the limbus and probably also in the palisades of Vogt in the adjacent conjunctiva.

While cells populating the corneal epithelium might seem to be always on the move, they paradoxically remain at all times firmly attached to the basement membrane and the cells around them. The epithelial adhesion is so strong that its weakest part is found in the tall columnar cells, which will rupture through the middle rather than losing adhesion to the basement membrane or attachment to overlying cells (Bergmanson and

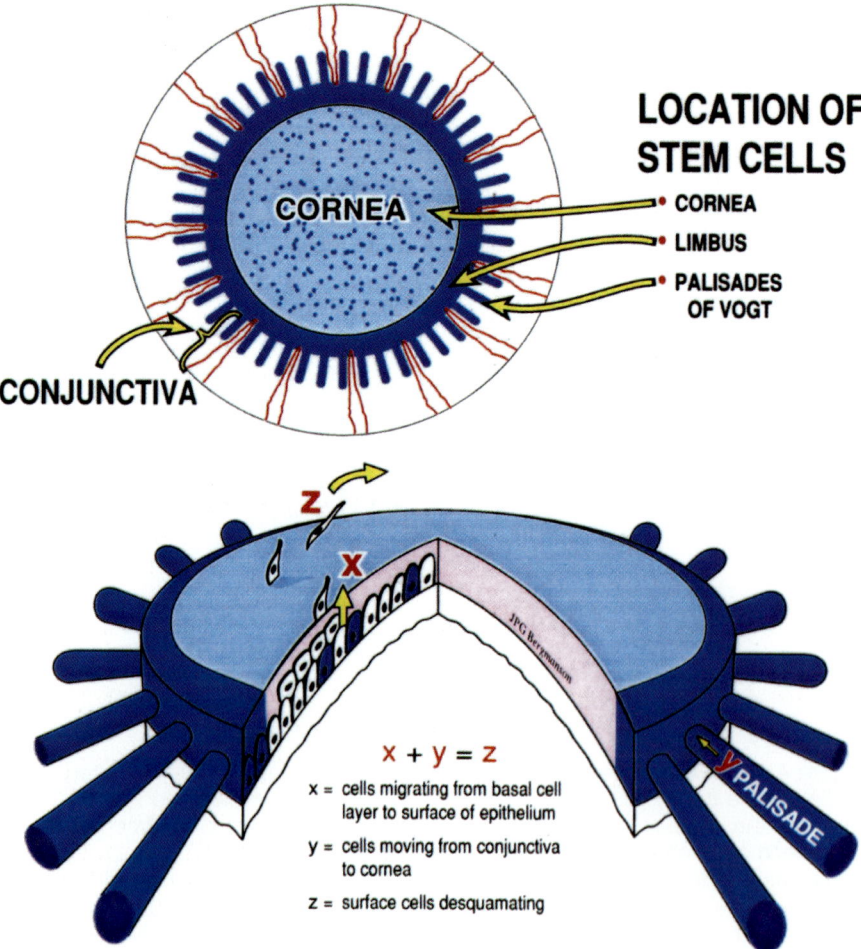

Figure 4.5 The X-Y-Z theory of epithelial cell proliferation, centripetal movement and desquamation (Reproduced from Bergmanson, 2000a)

Chu, 1982). This very strong adhesion is achieved through (1) a large number of hemidesmosomes found along the internal plasmalemma of the basal cell, which allow for the adhesion to the underlying cornea, and (2) a generous distribution of desmosomes formed between neighbouring cells, allowing for cell-to-cell adhesion. Further enhancement of the cell-to-cell adhesion is achieved through interdigitations between neighbouring cells. The combination of extensive intercellular interdigitations together with numerous desmosomes acting as 'spot welds', results in a very resilient structure that will, for instance, allow for a very vigorous rubbing of the eyes without abrasions occurring.

Other cell junctions in the epithelium are gap junctions and zonulae occludentes. The gap junctions are found between cells in all layers and they promote intercellular exchanges. The zonulae occludentes are only found in the superficial squamous cell layer and are there to provide an anterior fluid barrier. When this barrier is disturbed through trauma or inhibited by exposure to a hypotonic environment, fluid will enter the epithelium and accumulate between the cells. This is known as epithelial oedema, and is often clinically referred to as 'Sattler's veil' because of the significant visual effects of this condition (Krutsinger and Bergmanson, 1985).

The name of this layer ('epithelium') implies that it comprises only epithelial cells, but this is strictly not true. It is well known that the epithelium has a dense innervation. Most of the epithelial nerves are located deep in the basal cell layer. This is also the location of a third class of cells, Langerhans cells, that are normally resident in the epithelium. Langerhans cells are the outposts of the immune system. For more than 100 years they have been known to exist in the skin, but only relatively recently was it discovered that Langerhans cells also populate the cornea (Gillette et al., 1982). However, these cells are not found in the cornea in such a high density as occurs in the skin. The small body of the Langerhans cell is usually found deep in the epithelium, and projecting from its body are long rounded processes that span significant corneal distances. The Langerhans cells, like neurons, seem sensitive to environmental changes and challenges. Extended wear of contact lenses provokes an elevation of the number of Langerhans cells inhabiting the cornea (Hazlett et al., 1999) while UV-B radiation causes a net loss of Langerhans cells (Hill et al., 1994). White blood cells may, on occasions, be observed within the epithelium. However, they likely have been called upon in response to a challenge to the health of the cornea. Therefore, these cells should not be regarded as residents of the normal cornea, but rather as cells that are recruited when the integrity of the cornea is threatened.

Numerous tiny microvilli and microplicae form the surface of the epithelium and they have two proposed functions: (1) stabilization of the tear layer, and (2) increasing the surface area of the cornea. These cellular microprojections vary between species in shape and the pattern they form (Collin and Collin, 2000). They increase the absorption of nutrients such as oxygen but also help stabilize the tear film, or in aquatic animals, the mucous layer. Microvilli are mostly seen in corneas exposed to air, while microplicae are particularly well developed in marine animals (Collin and Collin, 2000).

Figure 4.6 is a schematic representation of some of the key structural and functional aspects of the epithelium.

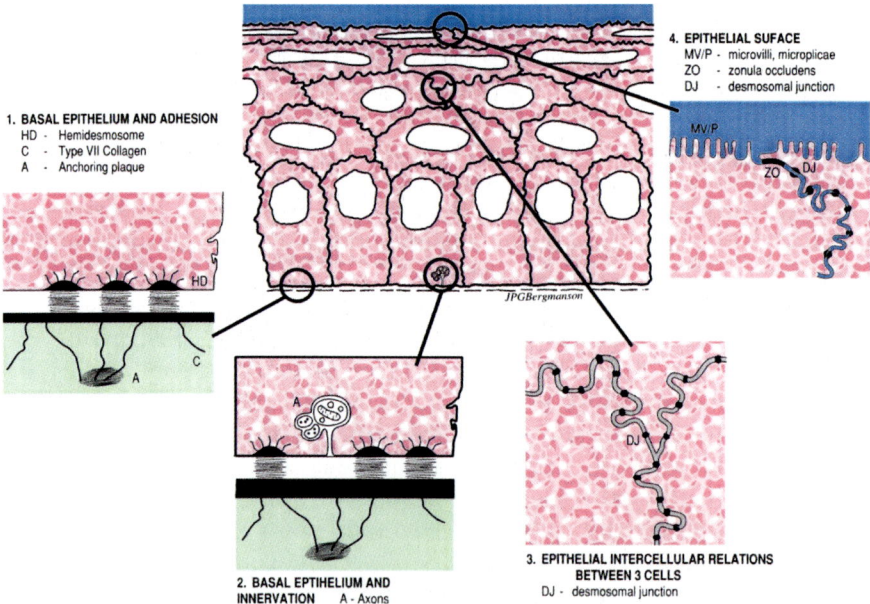

Figure 4.6 Key features of epithelial structure and function (Reproduced from Bergmanson, 2000a)

Anterior limiting lamina

The anterior limiting lamina (Bowman's membrane; ALL) measures $16.6 \pm 1.1 \, \mu m$ (Li *et al.*, 1997) and is modified stromal tissue. The ALL is acellular, except for the infrequent neural rami perforans, which are fine neural twigs penetrating this layer on their way to the epithelium. The ALL is formed by a dense network of fine, randomly oriented collagen Type I fibres, which are finer in cross-section than the underlying stromal collagen. The ALL provides attachments for the epithelial basement membrane by means of Type VII collagen fibres. These fibres originate from within the ALL and at their other end insert in the basement membrane (Figure 4.7). Thus, these fine fibrils are fused with the basement membrane anteriorly, while posteriorly they are held firm in anchoring plaques, which are found within the ground substance of the ALL. There are additional structures or proteins that contribute to the complex arrangement concerned with epithelial adhesion and these

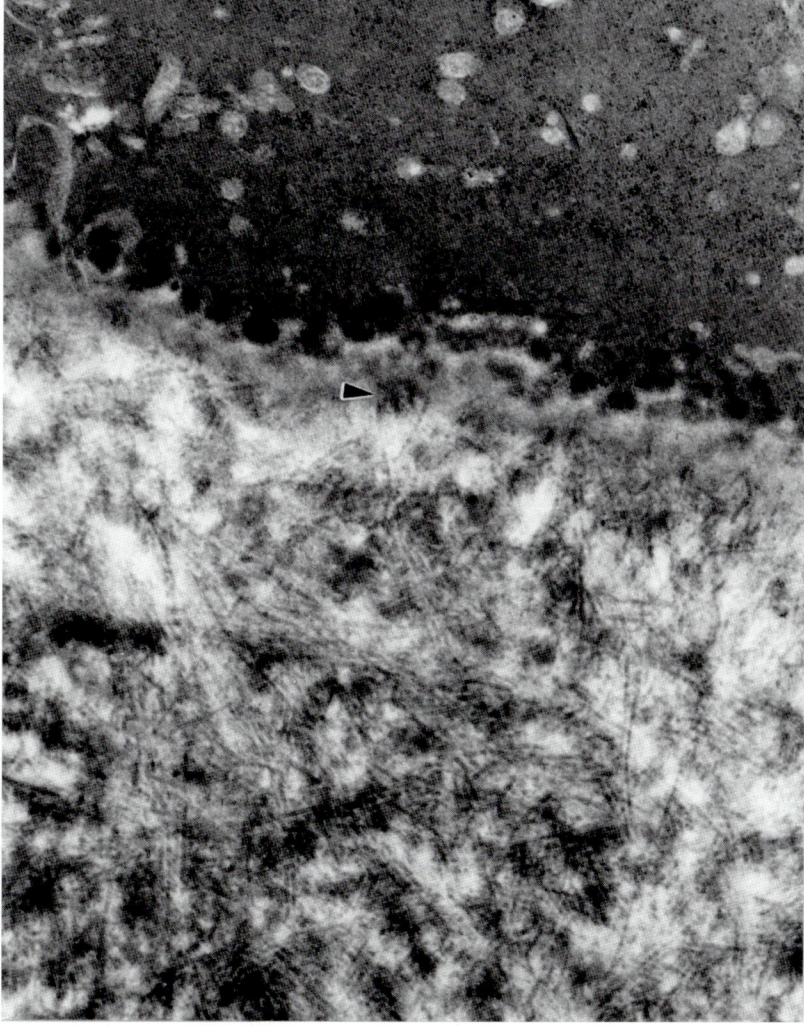

Figure 4.7 Flat section through the epithelium-stroma interface. Type VII collagen fibres (triangle) emanating from the anterior limiting lamina insert into the basement membrane. Rabbit. Electron micrograph, magnification ×14 100

include laminin and fibronectin. The ALL is strictly a corneal structure since it stops at the limbus. It is important to also realize that the ALL cannot regenerate. This is a dilemma that every cornea subjected to a photorefractive keratectomy (PRK) must overcome. The tissue in these instances must improvise to create a new interface between epithelium and stroma, to provide for the needed epithelial adhesion. It appears that the cornea does remarkably well in overcoming this obstacle, since few cases of recurrent erosion syndrome are reported following PRK.

Stroma

The stroma (substantia propria) constitutes 90% of the corneal thickness and is the structure that gives strength to the cornea. It is approximately 500 μm thick and is formed by collagen fibres, keratocytes and matrix. The collagen is primarily Type I, the most common collagen in the body. Type II collagen is primarily found in cultured embryonic cornea, and Type V and VI collagens have been reported in small quantities in the stroma. The collagen follows a highly organized pattern where the fibres are bundled together in lamellae. The collagen fibres in each lamella run parallel to each other. The lamellae, while remaining parallel to the surface of the eye, cross each other at various angles. The collagen in the stromal lamellae are of very similar calibre and are relatively uniformly spaced. As long as the fibres remain of uniform calibre and are not spaced further apart than $\lambda/2n$ (λ is the wavelength and n is the refractive index of the media), then the requirements for transparency are satisfied (Goldman and Benedek, 1967). Anteriorly, the stromal lamellae are slightly thinner and follow a more intertwined path (Figure 4.8), while posteriorly the lamellae are laid down flatter (Figure 4.9). This anatomical variation between anterior and posterior lamellae may partly explain the tendency of the cornea to swell from a posterior to an anterior direction.

The keratocyte is the principal cell of the stroma but other cells have been observed to be present in the normal stromal tissue. For instance, Kuwabara (1978) reported that small numbers of neutrophils, lympho-cytes, plasma cells and histocytes are present in the normal stroma. In addition, the anterior stroma harbours a plexus of unmyelinated nerve fibres and, thus, the stroma is also inhabited by both Schwann cells and neurons. Moller-Pedersen et al. (1994) calculated that the adult cornea contains 2.4 million keratocytes and that they exhibit a non-uniform topographic distribution throughout the stroma. The highest density of keratocytes is found anteriorly and from there the density declines in a posterior direction by as much as 30% (Moller-Pedersen and Ehlers, 1995; Petroll et al., 1995). A small increase in cell density was also noticed immediately anterior to the posterior limiting lamina. The keratocytes are

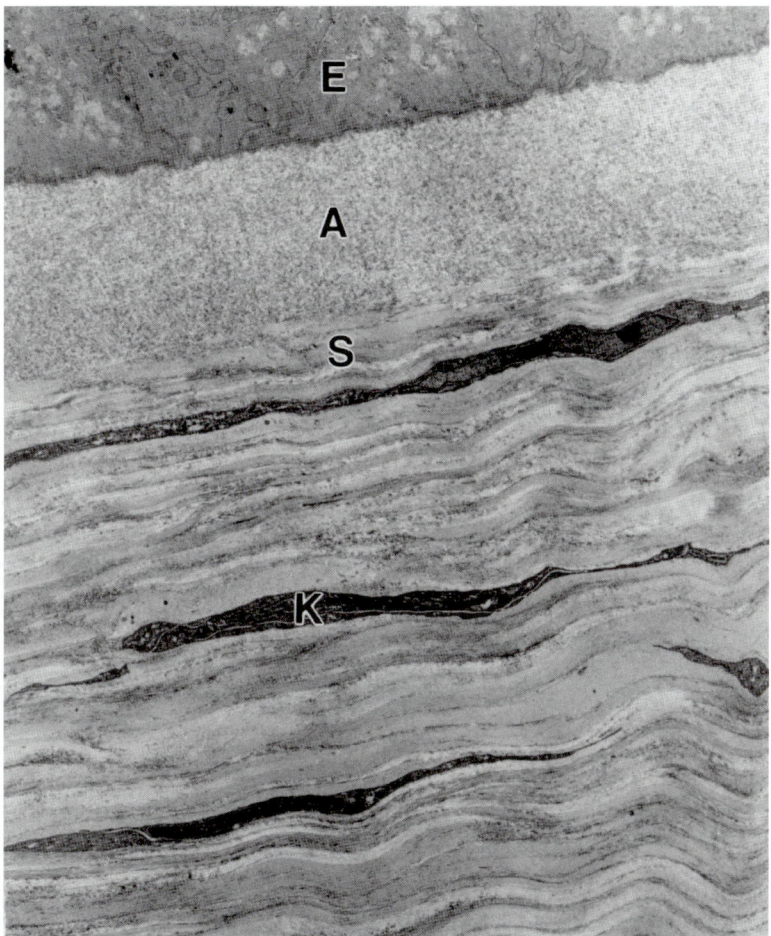

Figure 4.8 Transverse section through the anterior stroma. The anterior limiting lamina (A), sandwiched between the epithelium (E) and the stroma (S), is collagenous and acellular. Compared to the posterior stroma (see Figure 4.9), the anterior stroma contains more keratocytes (K) and the lamellae are thinner and more intertwined. Primate. Electron micrograph, magnification ×2700

primarily located between lamellae but their distribution in the stroma may not be as random as was first thought. Müller *et al.* (1995) reported that keratocytes were arranged in a regular clockwise spiralling pattern throughout the full stromal thickness.

Keratocytes are flattened to 'paper thin' proportions as they are lodged between the lamellae of the densely packed cornea. They have a spindle shape with long processes that extend horizontally. Vertical projections

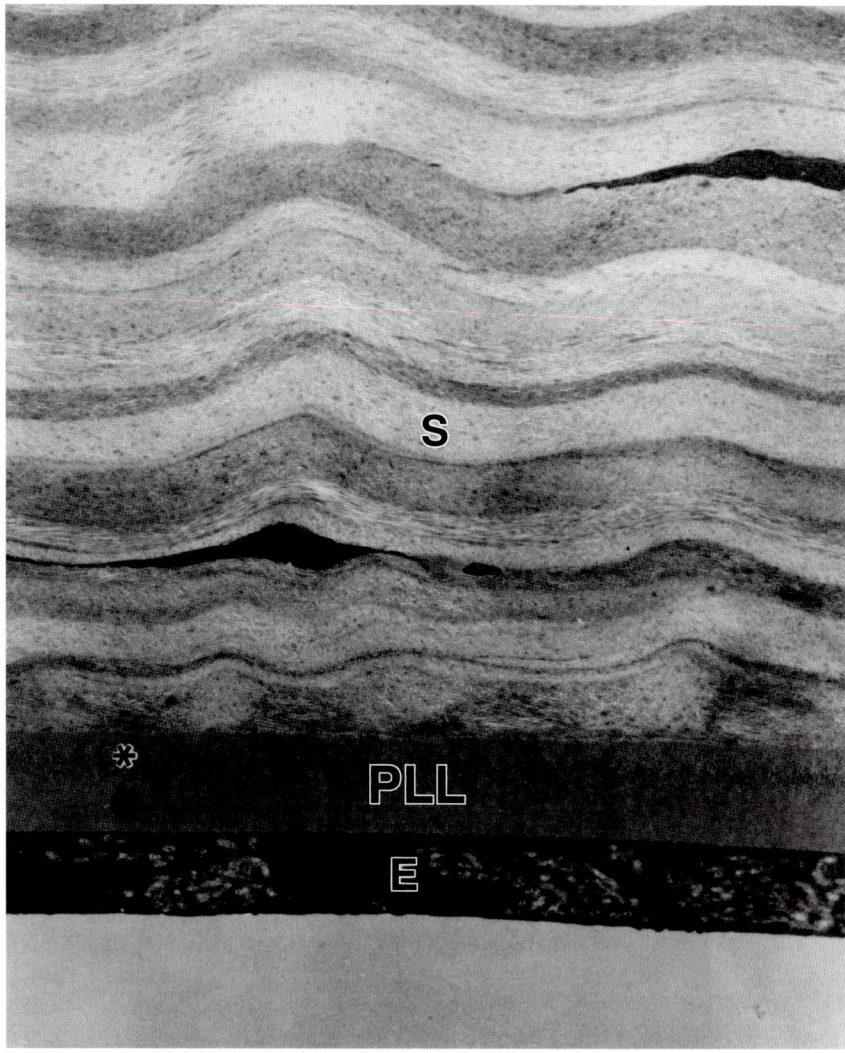

Figure 4.9 Transverse section through the posterior cornea. Compared to the anterior stroma (see Figure 4.8), the posterior stroma contains fewer keratocytes and the posterior stromal (S) lamellae are thicker and are laid down on top of each other in a more strict and orderly fashion. The endothelium (E) and its basement membrane, the posterior limiting lamina (PLL), are also present in this view. The anterior and posterior walls of the endothelium are parallel to each other as well as to the plane of the cornea. A large number of organelles can be observed in the endothelial cell. The PLL consists of the fetal banded portion (asterisk) and the postnatal non-banded portion (black dot). Primate. Electron micrograph, magnification ×3400

from cells crossing lamellae have been reported (Doughty *et al.*, in press). These have been called translamellar keratocytes (TLK) (Figure 4.10).

Almost 150 years ago in 1857, Claréus Hornhinnans observed that keratocytes form a closely linked network. More recently, a number of researchers have reported the existence of gap junctions between keratocytes (Müller *et al.*, 1995; Watsky, 1995; Doughty *et al.*, in press). Through the gap junctions the keratocytes can communicate across the cornea in both the horizontal direction and vertically (through TLKs).

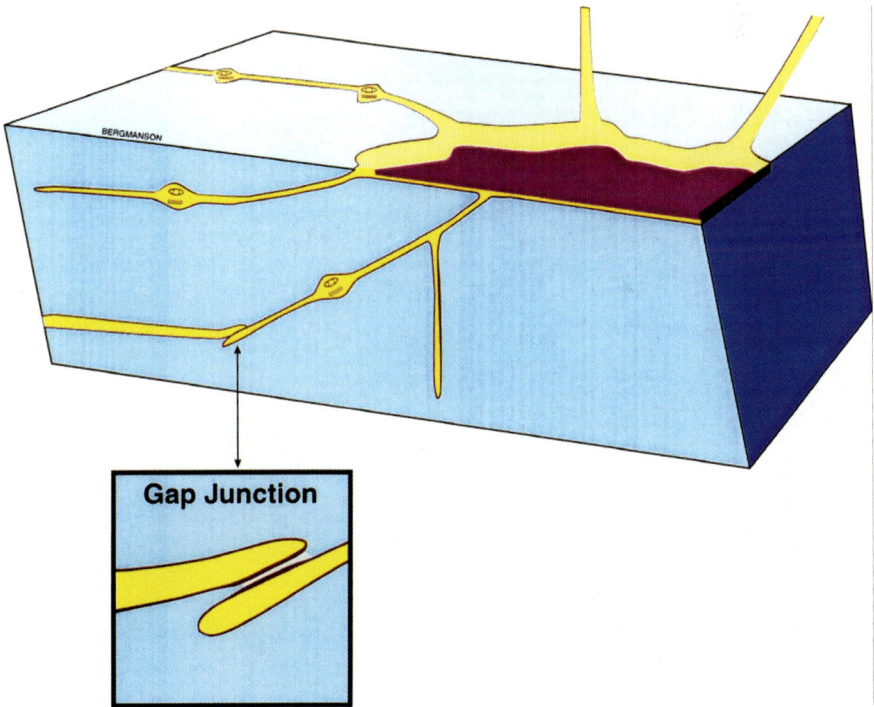

Figure 4.10 Schematic representation of a keratocyte showing a large nucleus and long cytoplasmic processes which communicate via gap junctions (Reproduced from Bergmanson, 2000a)

Keratocytes are a great deal more complex than previously thought. Mitochondria, rough endoplasmic reticulum, vesicles, Golgi fields and centrioles are organelles that have been reported to occur in these cells, often in significant numbers (Müller *et al.*, 1995; Doughty *et al.*, in press). The organelles are generally displaced peripheral to the nucleus because of the thinness of the cell (Figure 4.11). However, the existence of a generous number of organelles suggests a higher level of activity among

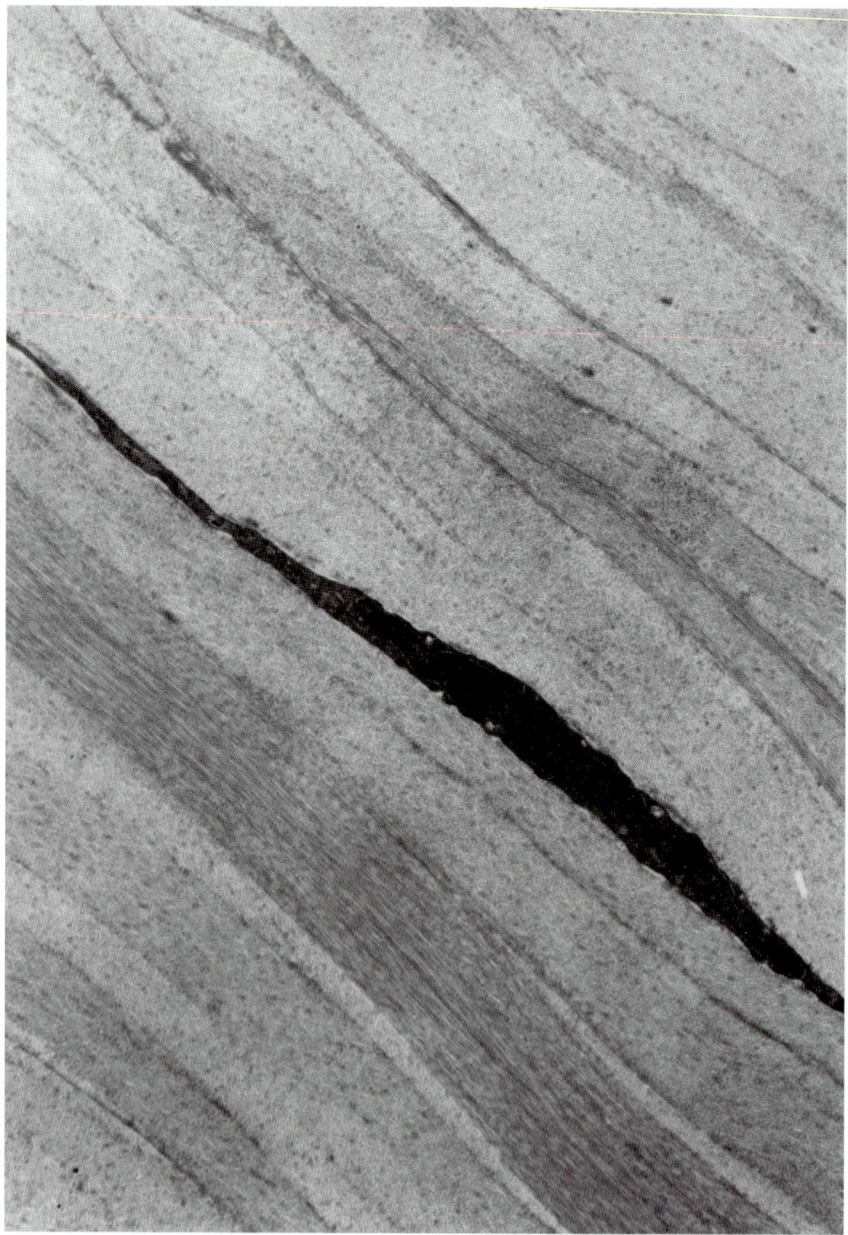

Figure 4.11 Transverse section through the mid-stroma. While lamellae cross each other at various angles, the collagen fibres within each lamella are all parallel to each other. A keratocyte (long, thin, dark, diagonally oriented feature in centre of frame) is sectioned through its nuclear portion. Cytoplasm around the nucleus is thin allowing the presence of few organelles, giving the false impression of an inactive cell. Primate. Electron micrograph, magnification ×5600

keratocytes than previously believed. This activity is at least partially devoted to exchanges with the surrounding matrix. Keratocytes are also an important reserve source of glycogen, which may be converted into glucose in stressful conditions. In transverse section, the keratocyte may appear as a quiet fixed cell, but in flat section, the keratocyte is truly revealed as a complex cell with multiple organelles; it also appears to be engaged in an intricate relationship with surrounding collagen lamellae. This close relationship between collagen fibres and keratocytes suggests that keratocytes may be involved in supporting lamellar stability. In other words, keratocytes help keep the different lamellae stable in the intended locations (Komai and Tatsuo, 1991; Müller *et al.*, 1995). In addition, it is also now known, thanks largely to laser refractive surgery, that the keratocyte plays a dominant role in corneal wound healing.

Posterior limiting lamina

The posterior limiting lamina (PLL, Descemet's membrane), measuring 3–20 µm thick, is truly a corneal layer, since it stops at the limbus. It is the basement membrane of the endothelium and it is also the thickest basement membrane in the body. It is continuously synthesized at a high rate throughout life by the endothelial cells (Figure 4.12). At birth, this membrane is approximately 3 µm thick and it grows at a rate of approximately 1 µm per decade (Johnson *et al.*, 1982). The most anterior portion is the oldest and it is also the least uniform. This is the fetal part of the membrane and it is known as the 'banded layer', whereas the postnatal part of the membrane is uniform in texture and is also the portion that thickens with age (Figure 4.9).

The adult peripheral PLL often shows pockets of local thickening known as Hassall–Henle warts. Similar irregularities in the PLL are sometimes noted centrally in the cornea and the condition is then known as corneal guttae (due to misuse of the Latin language, this condition is referred to as 'guttata' in some texts). Corneal guttae are usually self-limiting, but occasionally this condition, which is due to abnormal endothelial basement membrane synthesis, advances to affect the health of the endothelial cells (Bergmanson *et al.*, 1999). It then becomes known as Fuchs' endothelial dystrophy (Figure 4.13). As can be seen in Figure 4.13, the guttae cause extreme thinning of endothelial cells.

This condition leads to a compromise of endothelial pump function; however, as long as the endothelium maintains its coverage of the posterior cornea, uncontrolled oedema is avoided. The condition can progress to cause a loss of corneal transparency, whereby a penetrating keratoplasty may be necessary to restore vision. Certainly, Fuchs' endothelial dystrophy is one of the most common reasons for keratoplasty.

The PLL is a very resilient structure and it is the last corneal layer to give way in corneal melting. The anterior protrusion of the PLL that follows as a consequence of the erosion of the overlying stroma is termed a 'descemetocele'.

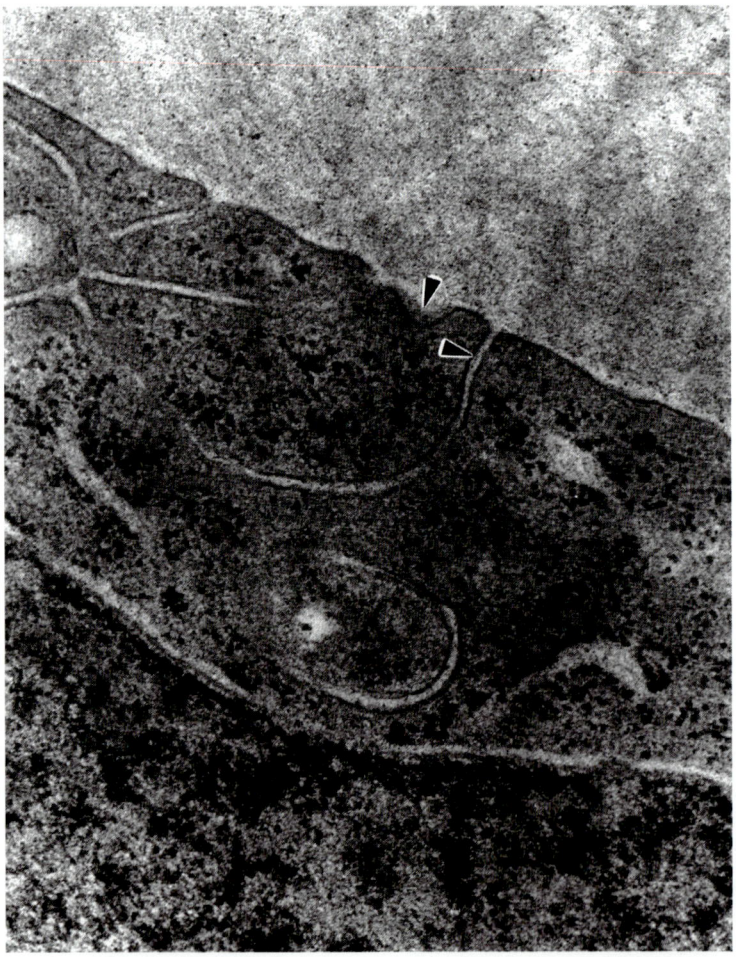

Figure 4.12 Transverse section through the interface between PLL and the endothelium. No hemidesmosomes are present but small particles (triangles) are noted between the PLL and the endothelium and in the narrow spacing between neighbouring cells. These particles are likely to be basement membrane material, which is continuously secreted by the endothelial cell. They appear to provide for the strong endothelial adhesion to the overlying cornea. Primate. Electron micrograph, magnification ×49 400

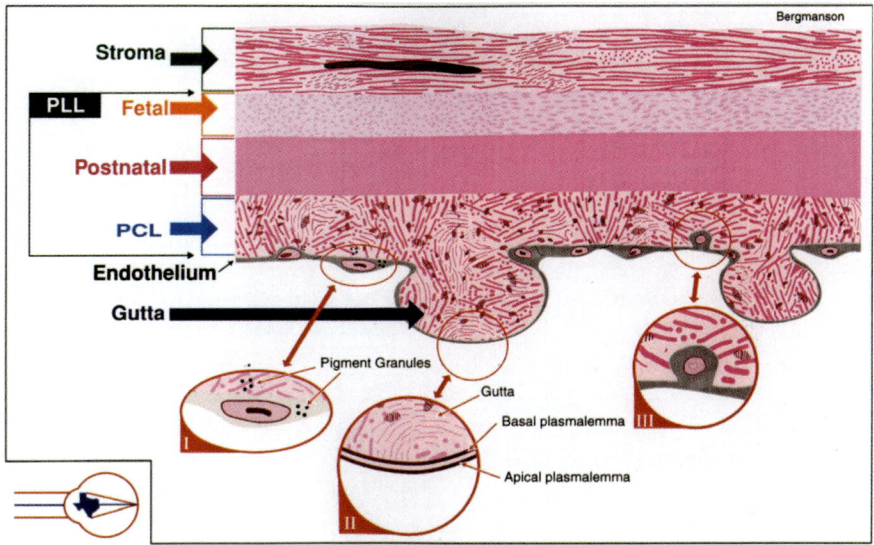

Figure 4.13 Schematic representation of the pathophysiological events in Fuchs' dystrophy (Reproduced from Bergmanson, 2000a).

Endothelium

A single layer of squamous epithelial cells forms the endothelium. These cells are 5 μm thick, with apical and basal sides strictly parallel to each other in the plane of the cornea. In a flat or coronal section, the endothelial cells are predominantly hexagonal in shape and measure approximately 18 μm across. When viewed clinically in this plane they form an extremely uniform mosaic. After birth, these cells do not normally reproduce, although it has been claimed that under special circumstances, such as injury, these cells may show mitosis. At the peripheral limit of the cornea, the endothelium is modified to form the trabecular meshes.

The function of the endothelium is to regulate the fluid entering the cornea from the aqueous. The endothelium accomplishes this by acting both as a 'leaky' fluid barrier and as a fluid pump, which removes fluid from the corneal tissue.

Since endothelial cells lose their ability to reproduce after birth, the cells resident on the posterior corneal surface must last a lifetime. Unfortunately, some cells will be lost over time. Therefore, there is a natural age-related decline in the number of corneal endothelial cells, as described in Table 4.2. There is a generous safety reserve to accommodate this loss. When an endothelial cell dies, the neighbouring cells spread out

Table 4.2 Endothelial cell density	
Age	*Cell density (cells/mm²)*
Birth	2987–5632 (Average: 4252–4425)
20–30 years	3000–3500
40–50 years	2500–3000
80 years	2000–2500
Functional limit	700–1000 (?)

laterally to cover the surface bared by the departing cell. However, disease or trauma may provoke excessive cell loss, which would interfere with normal endothelial function. With too few cells left, the individual endothelial cell will be unable to undergo lateral expansion sufficient to provide complete corneal coverage. Complete endothelial coverage of the posterior surface is essential for corneal transparency. In addition, the endothelial cell is actively involved in driving out fluid that naturally leaks into the cornea. However, with too few cells remaining, pumping activity sufficient to maintain a normal water balance will not be possible. Thus, excessive endothelial cell death has two effects that, in combination, lead to a loss of transparency through oedema and ultimately, corneal decompensation. The two effects are, first, the inability to provide full coverage of the posterior corneal surface and, second, the loss of pumping capacity. It is believed that the functional limit of the corneal endothelium is approximately 700–1000 cells/mm².

The endothelial cells contain a high density of mitochondria and rough endoplasmic reticulum (Figure 4.14). These organelles are hallmarks for metabolically active cells. A few scattered microvilli are present along the apical cell surface. The cells have, as mentioned above, very flat, parallel and linear apical and basal outlines, but their lateral walls show extensive interdigitations. These interdigitations increase the surface area of the cell and are one reason why the endothelial cell can expand laterally when this is called for.

Along the lateral sides, but near the apical side, junctional complexes are found. These junctional complexes contain zonulae occludentes (tight junctions), gap junctions and intermediate junctions. The zonulae occludentes, as elsewhere in the body, function as a fluid barrier.

However, research has shown that the zonulae occludentes in the epithelium do not wrap around the entire cell. This explains why the endothelium is a leaky membrane – allowing fluid to leak from the anterior chamber into the relatively dehydrated corneal stroma. The gap junctions found within these junctional complexes are concerned with intercellular communications, while the intermediate junctions (zonulae

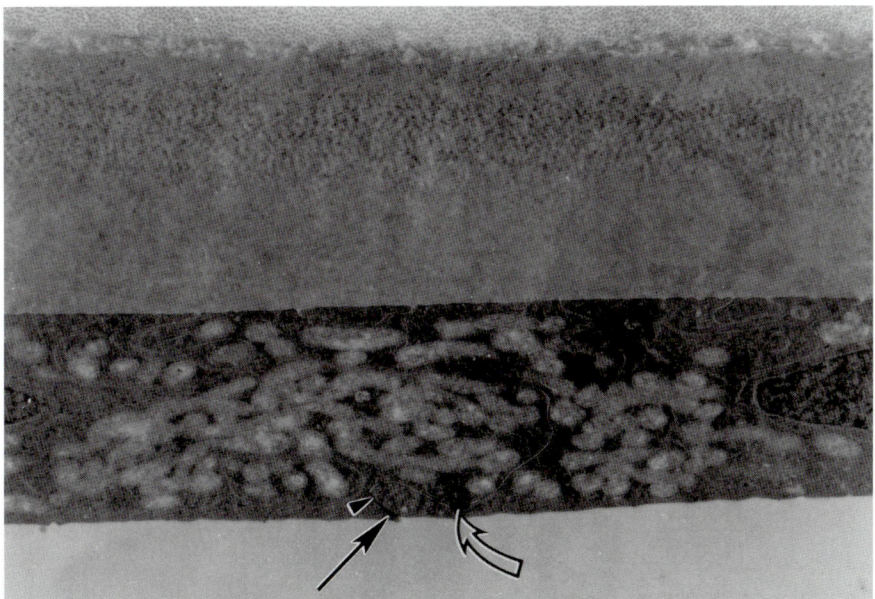

Figure 4.14 Transverse section through the endothelium and its accompanying basement membrane. The endothelial cell maintains a high count of organelles such as mitochondria and rough endoplasmic reticulum. A junctional complex between adjoining cells is evident and consists of a zonula occludens (arrow), a gap junction (triangle), and an intermediate junction (open arrow). Primate. Electron micrograph, magnification approximately ×9500

adherentes) provide cell-to-cell adhesion. These junctions are weaker than the desmosomes found in the epithelium, probably because the endothelium is not subjected to the physical forces the anterior surface may be facing. Table 4.3 provides a summary of the various junctional complexes observed in the corneal epithelium and endothelium.

Corneal nerves

The cornea has a rich supply of sensory nerve fibres, and in the human cornea no nerve fibres are of autonomic origin. The small nerves derive

Table 4.3 Corneal cell junctions		
Junction	*Epithelium*	*Endothelium*
Zonulae occludentes	Present	Present
Zonulae adherentes/intermediate junction	Absent	Present
Maculae adherentes/desmosomes	Present	Absent
Hemidesmosomes	Present	Absent
Gap junctions	Present	Present
Significant basement membrane secretion	Absent	Present

primarily from the long ciliary nerves, but also some from the short ciliary nerves enter the cornea near the limbus at the mid-stromal level. About 1.5 mm into the cornea, these fibres, if myelinated, lose their myelinated sheath since myelination is opaque and will obscure vision. The unmyelinated fibres split and further divide into smaller branches, which can cross two-thirds of the cornea (Figure 4.16). These nerves may be seen clinically. Other nerve fibres of similar origin follow a similar route, but in the epithelium.

The epithelial nerves lack the Schwann cell wrapping that fibres have in the stroma, and therefore nerve fibres are 'naked' in the epithelium. A group of four axons – two of which show terminal swelling – are shown in Figure 4.15. The close association between axons and epithelial cells suggests that the epithelium has taken over the function of the Schwann cell (Figure 4.17). There appears to be little communication between the epithelial and stromal nerve plexi. Single traversing rami perforantes have been noted, but are not common. It has been proposed that corneal nerves utilize peptidergic as well as acetylcholine neurotransmitters (Müeller *et al.*, 1996).

Stromal nerve fibres terminate usually within 25 µm of the epithelium (Figure 4.18). Therefore, like the epithelial nerves, they are positioned to respond to external stimuli. Very few axons ascend to reach the surface cells of the cornea. This arrangement explains why the epithelial trauma threshold is lower than the corneal touch threshold (Millodot and O'Leary, 1981). The epithelial nerve plexus is denser than the stromal plexus in a ratio of two to one (Bergmanson, 1988).

The corneal nerves have two main functions. First, they serve a protective role by mediating an aversion reflex in response to touch and other noxious stimuli. Second, corneal nerves have a trophic function – loss of corneal nerves leads to neuroparalytic keratitis.

Corneal sensitivity is measured as its touch threshold, which varies according to location (Table 4.4). Touch is one of five sensory modalities (pain, touch, heat, cold, pressure). The corneal touch threshold has proven

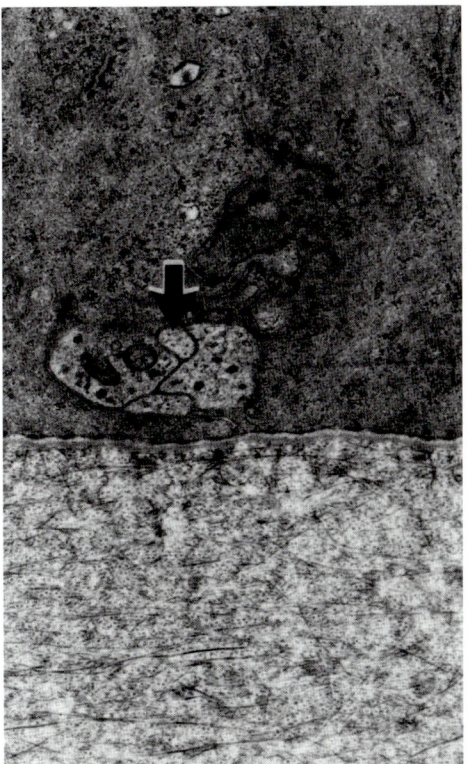

Figure 4.15 Epithelial innervation. Four axons (arrow) are located in an infolding of the basal cell internal plasmalemma. The two larger axons are at terminal level. Primate. Electron micrograph, magnification ×11 200

to be a very sensitive measure of corneal health, and the cornea being perhaps the most sensitive organ in the body. Particularly, this has been shown to be a useful measurement in contact lens wear, where the touch threshold may increase by over 100% when a non-gas permeable polymethyl methacrylate (PMMA) lens is worn (Millodot, 1976b). The instrument used for this purpose is known as a corneal aesthesiometer;

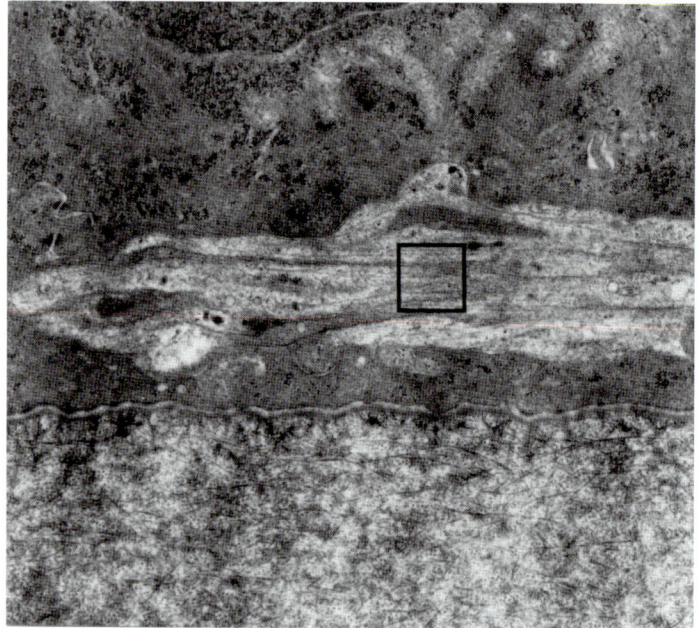

Figure 4.16 Longitudinal section through epithelial nerve, showing a group of axons (square) running deep within a basal cell and parallel to the basement membrane. Primate. Electron micrograph, magnification ×22 100

however, interpretation of data is often difficult due to significant individual variation, relating primarily to iris colour, and to differences among races (Millodot, 1976a) (Table 4.5).

Effects of contact lens wear on the corneal microstructure

Contact lenses can have an effect upon all major corneal structures – the epithelium, stroma and endothelium. This is not surprising, since the cornea is the tissue onto which the lens is directly placed. The epithelium is often the first region to react, or, indeed, the origin of a complication manifesting itself elsewhere in the cornea, as in hypoxia-induced oedema.

Many of the effects that a contact lens may have on the cornea can be observed clinically using the slit lamp. In the case of surface defects, fluorescein sodium chloride is often used to highlight the disturbance. But this staining technique does not reveal what is happening at a cellular

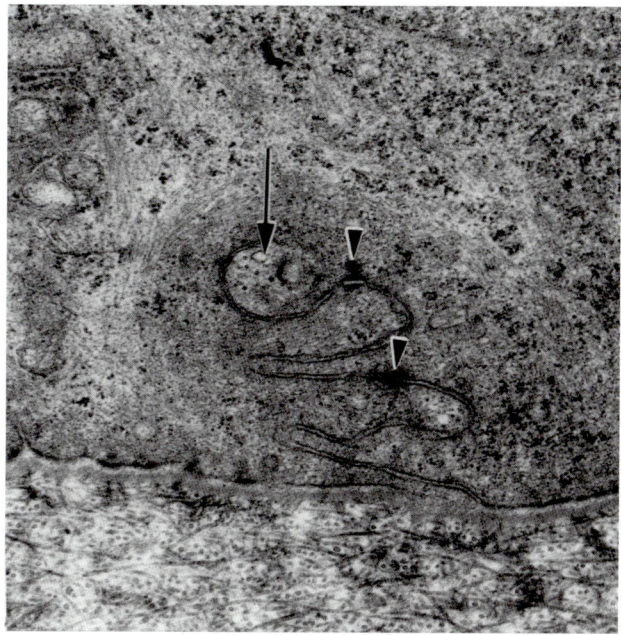

Figure 4.17 Epithelial-neural relations. A single axon (arrow) is observed deep in an epithelial infolding. In the epithelium the axon lacks its customary Schwann cell wrapping. The infolding shows two desmosomes (triangles). Primate. Electron micrograph, magnification ×22 100

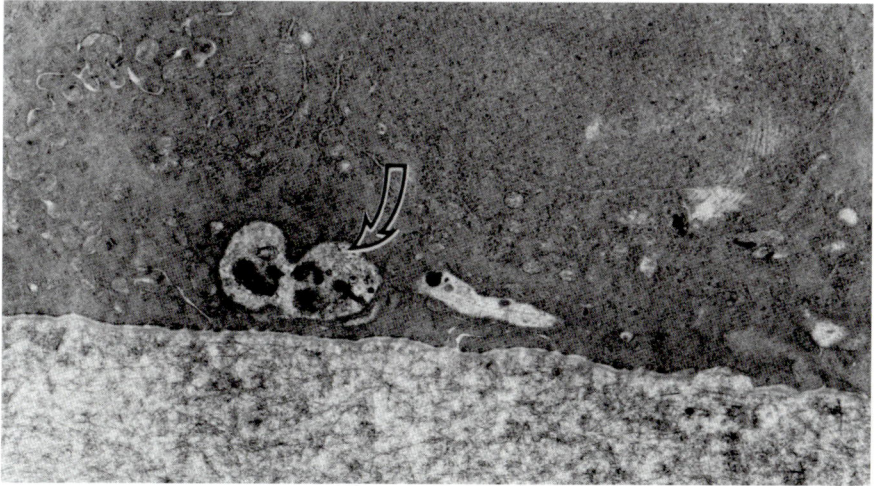

Figure 4.18 An epithelial nerve terminal (arrow) with two consecutive varicosities. The axon varicosities are adjacent to the basal plasmalemma of a basal cell and contain vesicles and mitochondria. Primate. Electron micrograph, magnification approximately ×17 000

Table 4.4 Approximate regional corneal touch thresholds (mg/mm^2)	
Corneal apex	20
Corneal periphery	40
Corneal conjunctiva	70–200 (peaks in fornix)
Lid margin	>20

level. Histopathological techniques allow such observations to be made. Below is a brief description of what may occur histopathologically in contact lens-wearing corneas. More complete reviews are available in the literature (see Bergmanson and Chu, 1982; Bergmanson *et al.*, 1985; Bergmanson, 1992, 1998, 2000b).

Abrasion and punctate staining

Punctate staining (sometimes called stippling), which is frequently observed in contact lens wearers, refers to a loss of epithelial cells. To be

Table 4.5 Ethnic and racial eye colour corneal touch thresholds (mg/mm^2)		
Race	*Eye colour*	*Mean corneal touch threshold*
Caucasian	Blue	14
	Hazel	16
	Green	22
	Brown	30
Indian	Dark brown	47
African	Dark brown	62
Chinese	Dark brown	65

Source: Millodot, 1976a.

seen clinically, a small group of maybe 5 to 10 cells needs to dislodge together. Gaps that form in the surface – which are left by isolated desquamating cells as occurs during the natural epithelial cell turnover – would be too minute to see with a slit lamp during routine corneal examination. The loss of a small group of cells normally does not lead to symptomatology. This is probably due to the fact that the trauma threshold for the epithelium is less than the touch sensitivity threshold (Millodot and O'Leary, 1981), which in turn is probably due to the fact that most nerve endings are deep in the basal cell layer with only a sparse innervation of the superficial epithelial layers.

Punctate staining is normally not regarded as too worrisome in contact lens wearers, but when these dot-like defects coalesce to larger areas clinical action is required. By definition this is an abrasion, which may be superficial or deep. Research has shown that a contact lens is not capable of inflicting injury deeper than the epithelial basement membrane (Bergmanson and Chu, 1982). The gentle scraping to debride the epithelium in preparation for photorefractive keratectomy (PRK) achieves the same result. Depending on the size of the abrasion, the epithelium will need 1–4 days to again provide stromal coverage. However, it will take a few days more for the cells to re-establish normal cell-to-cell contacts (McCartney and Cantu-Crouch, 1992). Therefore, it would be prudent in contact lens wearers with abrasions to wait until there has been no staining detected for one or two days before resuming lens wear.

Epithelial thinning

Epithelial thinning is not often discussed among clinicians and this probably has to do with the fact that it is a difficult condition to observe clinically. Its existence has been shown in clinical contact lens populations (Holden et al., 1985) and in animal studies (Bergmanson et al., 1985) (Figure 4.19). Several different scenarios may lead to epithelial thinning. Firstly, the mere presence of a lens inhibits epithelial mitosis in the central cornea (Ren et al., 1999; Ladage et al., 2000) and with cell shedding exceeding reproduction, the epithelium is bound to become thinner. The physical weight and tension of the lid may compress the mouldable epithelium to become more flattened (Bergmanson et al., 1985). For instance, the tall columnar cells may become cuboidal. Furthermore, a lack of nutritious tears may lead to premature sloughing and consequent epithelial thinning (Bergmanson and Wilson, 1989). A combination of all these above factors may contribute to the epithelial thinning, which is seen in successful extended-wear patients (Holden et al., 1985).

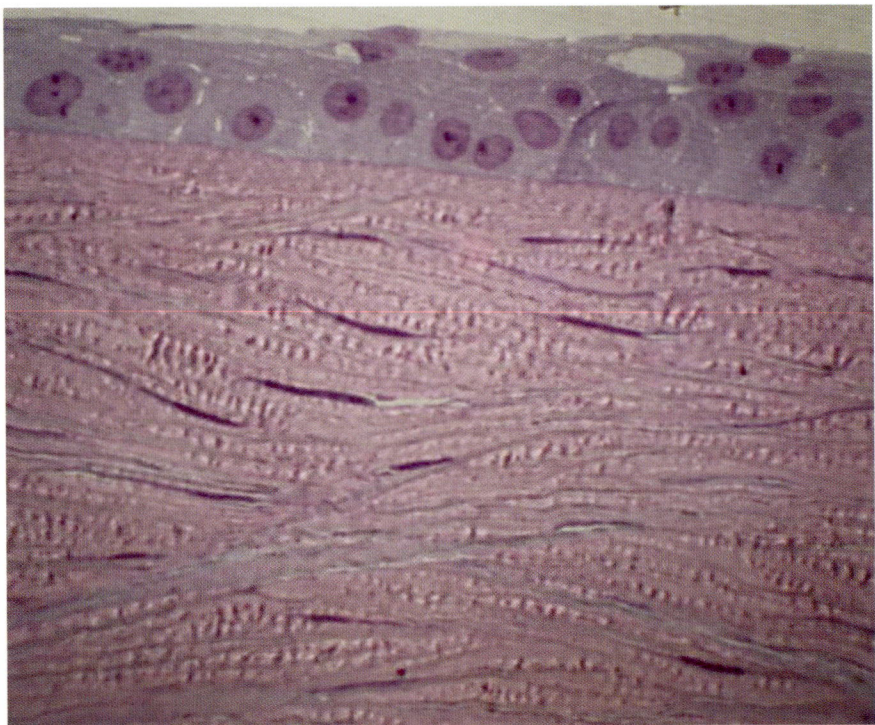

Figure 4.19 Light micrograph showing epithelial thinning in a cornea of a rhesus monkey that wore a rigid lens for 24 hours. The epithelium has a reduced number of cell layers. Compounding the thinning effect is a general flattening of cells. For instance, the columnar basal cells are approximately cuboidal. Mild epithelial oedema is manifested by small spaces around the cells and these spaces have probably appeared as a result of losing the fluid barrier located among the surface squamous cells. Toluidine blue. Magnification approximately ×300

Epithelial oedema

The aetiology of epithelial oedema is two-fold. Firstly, epithelial oedema follows traumatic loss of surface epithelial cells. The fluid barrier (zonula occludens) is found between surface epithelial cells and, thus, when it is removed, fluid may move in. Since the cells are tightly fitted and attach snugly together, the oedema may not occur instantly nor be widespread. Animal studies have demonstrated the coexistence of epithelial oedema and thinning following periods of rigid lens wear (Figure 4.20). Secondly, epithelial oedema follows hypotonic ocular exposure, which has an inhibiting effect on the fluid barrier.

The flare seen in and around abrasions is epithelial oedema. Histopathological evaluation of corneas following hypotonic exposure demonstrates that the oedema is extracellular and always of full epithelial thickness (Krutsinger and Bergmanson, 1985). Reflex tears are of low tonicity and may also provoke epithelial oedema, for instance during adaptation to rigid lenses (Schoessler and Lowther, 1971).

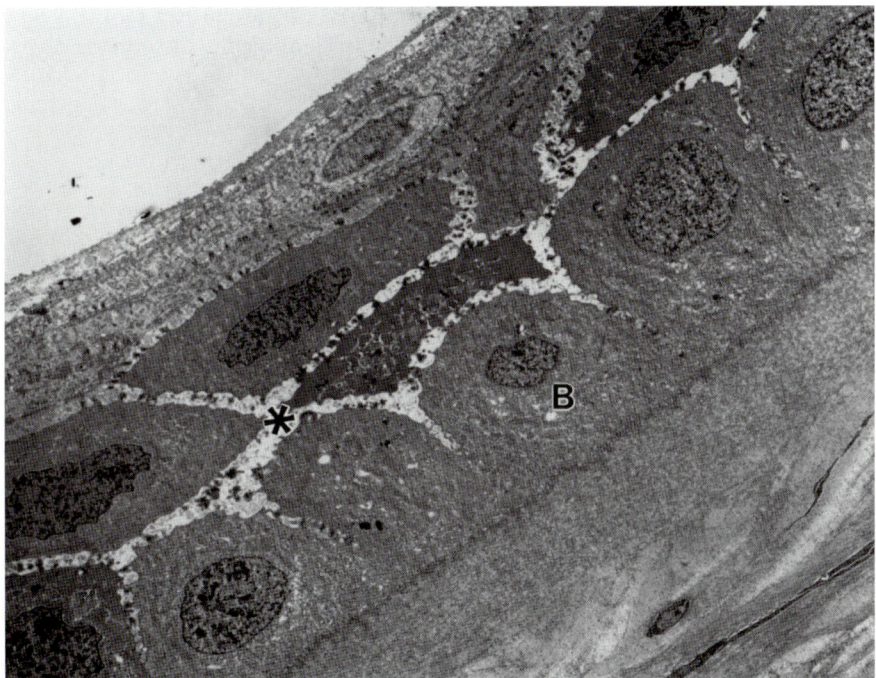

Figure 4.20 Transmission electron micrograph of the epithelium after 24 hours of wear of a hard contact lens in a rhesus monkey. This transverse section illustrates epithelial thinning and oedema. Epithelial thinning is largely due to partial collapse of cellular shape; the tall columnar basal cells (B) have become almost cuboidal in shape. The epithelial oedema (asterisk) is intercellular with little or no fluid within the cells. Magnification ×5000

Contaminated low tonicity water, such as that which may be found in a hot tub, has an association with contracting an acanthamoeba keratitis. The acanthamoebas may use the spaces created between cells by the oedematous state to gain entry to the cornea. This scenario is possible in both contact lens wearers and non-lens wearers.

Recent work has shown that debris trapped between a silicon hydrogel lens and the eye can indent the epithelial surface (Pritchard *et al.*, 2000).

This debris, which is referred to as 'mucin balls' or 'lipid plugs', appears only to leave an imprint on the delicate and mouldable epithelial surface, but probably does not damage the fluid barrier.

An interesting finding is that extended contact lens wear leads to an elevation of the number of Langerhans cells resident in the central cornea (Hazlett *et al.*, 1999). Langerhans cells are important cells in the immune response in the skin and the cornea. In the cornea they are found fixed among the basal cells, sending their long slender processes across large areas. It has been proposed that this cellular reorganization could assist the eye in responding more promptly to insults, making the cornea more prone to an inflammatory reaction.

Stroma

The major cell of the stroma, the keratocyte, may be affected by contact lens wear. Under more hypoxic conditions keratocytes may react adversely (Bergmanson and Chu, 1982). Loss of epithelial coverage, as in a deep abrasion, is known to eliminate keratocytes in superficial stroma (Dohlman *et al.*, 1968; Campos *et al.*, 1994; You *et al.*, 1995), but they will later return (You *et al.*, 1995). This shows that keratocytes are very sensitive cells that react to changes in the environment. Slight stromal thinning was reported in long-term extended-wear patients (Holden *et al.*, 1985), and perhaps this may be explained by a loss of keratocytes.

The stromal lamellar architecture shows a difference between the anterior and posterior stroma. The lamellae in the anterior stroma tend to be more intertwined, while those in the posterior stroma are simply laid down on top of each other but at varying angles. This may be a structural factor in explaining the propensity for the stroma to first become oedematous posteriorly.

Interestingly, when the stroma becomes oedematous, it does not manifest itself as a universal widening of the gap between collagen fibres. Instead the fluid build-up is primarily between the lamellae and around keratocytes (Bergmanson and Chu, 1982) (Figure 4.21). Although some intralamellar oedema may be present, the most striking feature in stromal swelling is the pooling of fluid around keratocytes, which possibly leads to lamellar separation.

Endothelium

Since Schoessler and Woloschak (1981) reported endothelial polymegethism (variation in cell size) as a consequence of contact lens wear, a considerable amount of work has been conducted on this topic. Other

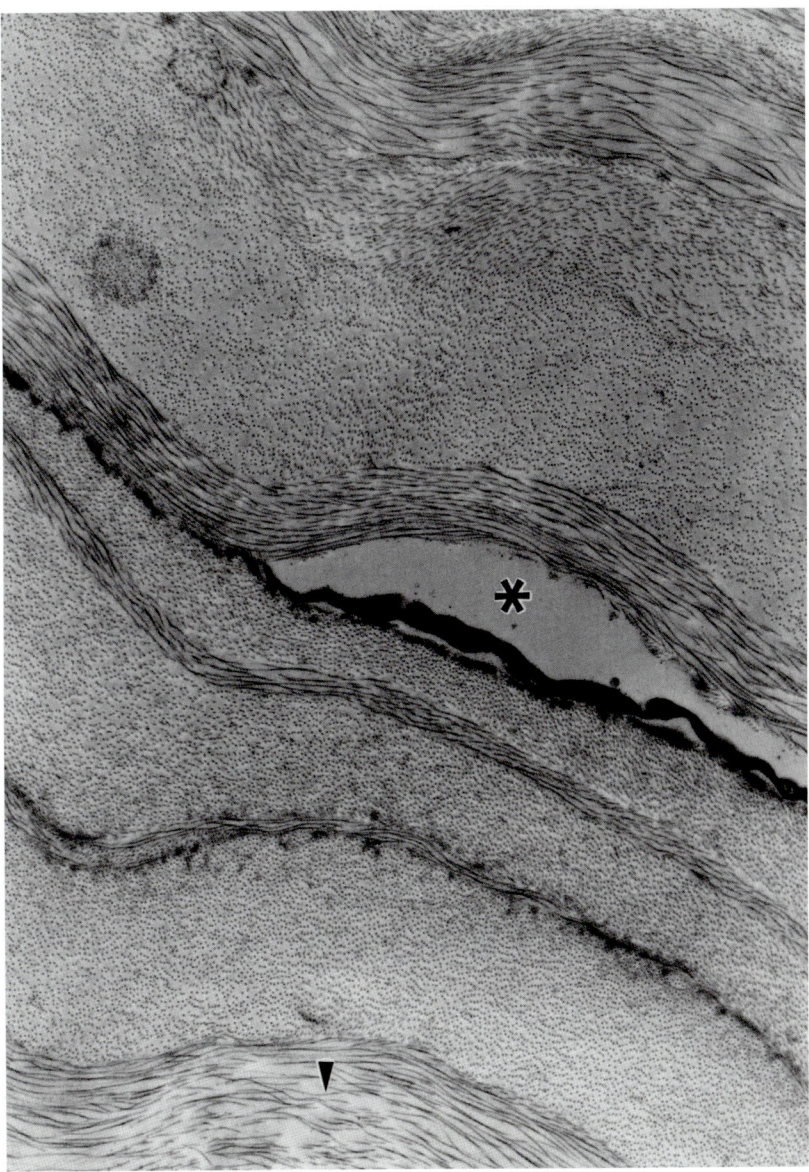

Figure 4.21 Stromal oedema is most conspicuous around keratocytes and between lamellae, where pooling (asterisk) may be present. Intralamellar swelling (triangle) is also evident in places. Primate. Electron micrograph. Magnification ×8500

features of the endothelium that have been studied include cell density, pleomorphism (variation in cell shape) and polygonality (variation in the number of cell sides) (Figure 4.22). A comprehensive review of this clinical condition is not within the scope of this chapter but several are available in the literature (see Doughty, 1989; Bergmanson, 1992; Efron, 1999).

Histopathological examination of polymegethous human endothelia has revealed that cells contain normal, healthy-appearing organelles and, therefore, are presumably functioning in a normal manner (Bergmanson, 1992). However, in this study it was observed that the lateral sides had adopted an oblique instead of a primarily straight anterior–posterior

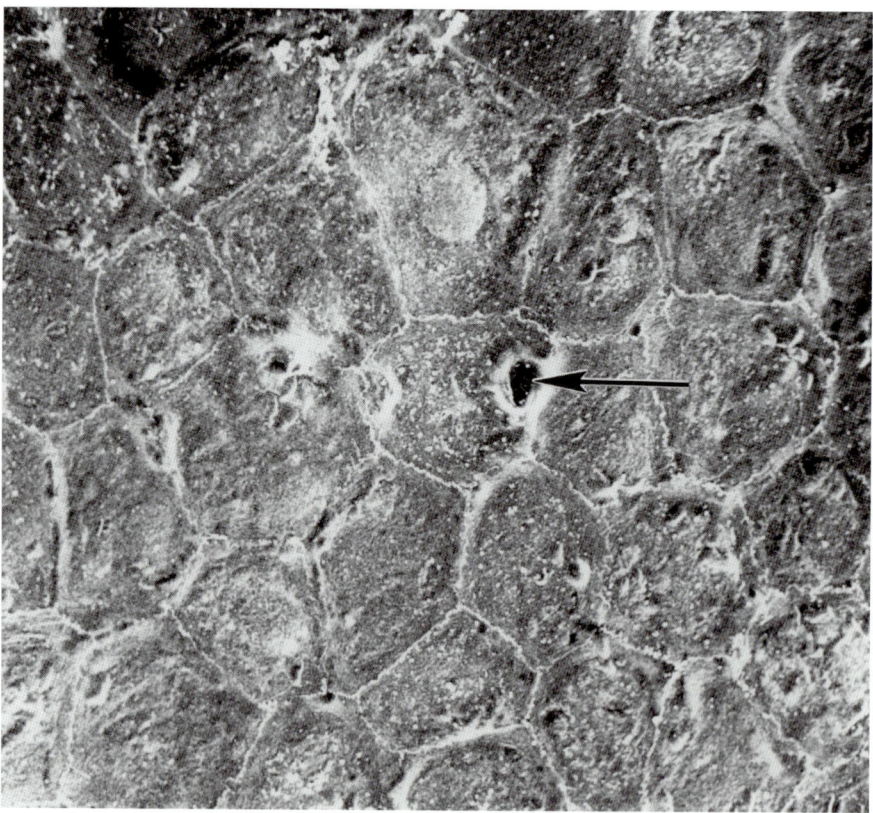

Figure 4.22 Scanning electron micrograph depicting the effect of daily wear aphakic hydrogel lens wear in a 66-year-old person. The intercellular variation in size (coefficient of variation of cell size = 0.31), polygonality and shape are noticeable. An intercellular oedematous space (arrow) has opened up towards the anterior chamber. Magnification approximately ×800 (Reproduced with permission from Bergmanson, 1992)

orientation (Figure 4.23). This observation allowed a different interpretation of the clinical picture obtained through specular endothelial
viewing, which is only a two-dimensional image of the interface between
the anterior chamber and the endothelium. In other words, only the
posterior (apical) wall of the endothelial cell is observed and this does not
facilitate a ready appreciation of the actual three-dimensional cell
configuration. Indeed, the observations of the slanted lateral sides is
suggested as a possible explanation of the polymegethism, whereby cells
with large posterior apical sides could have small basal (anterior) sides
and vice versa. Thus, cells rearranged their sides three-dimensionally to

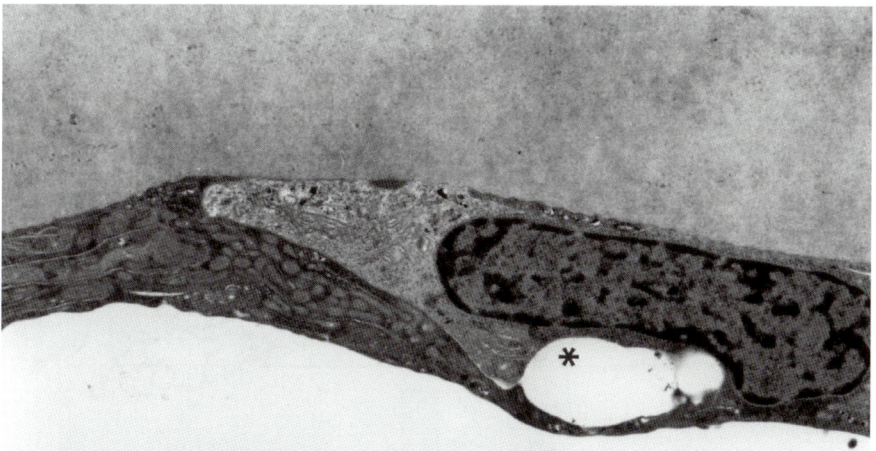

Figure 4.23 Transmission electron micrograph of the endothelium following
daily wear of an aphakic hydrogel lens in a 66-year-old person (same as
previous page). This transverse section demonstrates the oblique reorientation
of the lateral sides of the endothelial cells. An intercellular oedematous
space (asterisk) has formed between two neighbouring cells. Magnification
approximately ×18 000 (Reproduced with permission from Bergmanson, 1992)

a change in the environment but did not shrink or become bloated (Figure
4.24). If this turns out to be true, then polymegethism may not be a
disturbing threat to the cell and, therefore, not of major concern to the
clinician.

If there is a functional consequence from developing contact lens-
induced polymegethism, it has yet to be demonstrated. It has been
suggested that the corneal deswelling function is negatively affected
(Polse *et al.*, 1990). However, other studies have been unable to detect a
functional deficit in the polymegethous endothelium (Carlson *et al.*, 1988;
Bourne *et al.*, 1999). Now, two decades after the initial discovery, the

clinical calamity that contact lens-induced polymegethism would bring about – as predicted by some researchers – has yet to be realized. Although some functional deficit associated with this condition may still be uncovered, it seems increasingly unlikely that it will be one of clinical consequence.

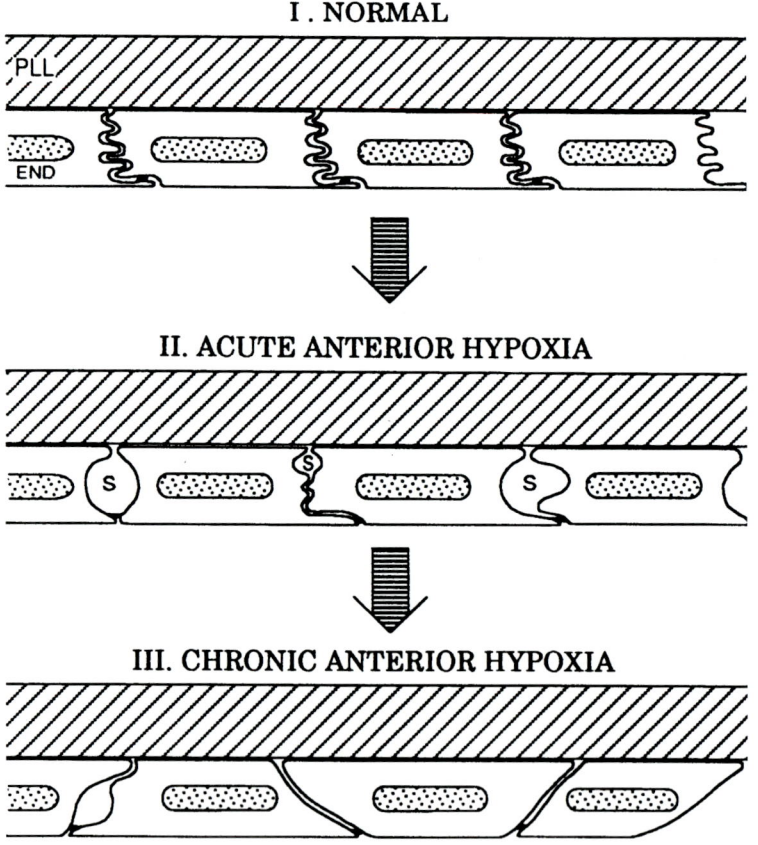

Figure 4.24 Hypothesis of the evolution of contact lens-induced endothelial polymegethism. I: The lateral sides of the normal endothelial cell are highly interdigitated and approximately perpendicular to the plane of the cornea. II: Potential spaces between the lateral sides of adjacent cells expand in response to acute hypoxic stress. The stretching of the lateral sides unfolds the interdigitations. III: The straightened lateral sides have adopted an oblique orientation relative to the plane of the cornea. This allows for a cell with a large posterior surface to have a small anterior surface, or vice versa. Thus, cellular volume may be unchanged and the endothelium, as a consequence, may not be occupied by cells that randomly became bloated or dwarfed by a hypoxic stimulus (Reproduced with permission from Bergmanson, 1992)

The methodology by which data are collected to quantify polymegethism has also been questioned (Doughty, 1989, 1990; Hirsch *et al.*, 1989). In some studies, the sample used to state the condition of 500 000 cells is as small as 50–75 cells, and only one out of the six sides that form the cells is considered. Perhaps too many assumptions have been made in efforts to understand contact lens-induced polymegethism.

One aspect of endothelial function relating to contact lens wear that appears to have been demonstrated unequivocally, is that contact lens wear does not lead to an accelerated decline in cell density beyond that seen in ageing (Hirst *et al.*, 1984; Holden *et al.*, 1985; MacRae *et al.*, 1986).

Conclusions

Through a combination of light and electron microscopic studies of the normal cornea and the cornea that has been challenged by contact lens wear, it has been possible to explain various clinical phenomena that clinicians have observed with the slit lamp. Perhaps more importantly, these techniques have provided supplementary information concerning the effects of contact lens wear on the cornea that cannot be detected clinically. An example of a phenomenon revealed by electron microscopy that perhaps ought to be of concern to contact lens practitioners is the ultrastructural decompensation that takes place in the epithelium. Conversely, electron microscopic evaluation of endothelial polymegethism induced by contact lens wear suggests that this change may be a harmless physiological adaptation rather than potentially devastating pathological change.

Emerging technologies such as confocal microscopy, nuclear magnetic resonance imaging and molecular biology will not diminish the role of the electron microscope as a tool for studying the cornea. To the contrary, it is certain that all of these technologies will supplement each other in assisting researchers and eye care practitioners to develop an ever-increasing body of knowledge to underpin our understanding of clinical matters relating to contact lens wear. Such ongoing research will also assist the ophthalmic industry in producing even better and safer contact lenses – and indeed other extraocular and intraocular appliances – for the betterment of the visual welfare of our patients.

Acknowledgements

I am grateful for the diligent work of William Tran and Danielle Robertson, who provided generous assistance in producing this manuscript.

References

Albert, D. M. and Edwards, D. D. (eds) (1996) Discovering the anatomy of the eye. In *The History of Ophthalmology*, pp. 47–63, Blackwell Science.

Bennett, A. G. and Rabbetts, R. B. (1998) The schematic eye. In *Clinical Visual Optics*, pp. 207–228, Butterworth-Heinemann.

Bergmanson, J. P. G. (1981) Corneal epithelial mitosis. A possible explanation to corneal stippling. *Contacto*, **25**, 19–22.

Bergmanson, J. P. G. (1988) The central corneal innervation in primates. *Am. J. Optom. Physiol. Optics*, **65**, 56P.

Bergmanson, J. P. G. (1992) Histopathological analysis of corneal endothelial polymegethism. *Cornea*, **11**, 133–142.

Bergmanson, J. P. G. (2000a) *Clinical Ocular Anatomy and Physiology*, 8th edn, Texas Eye Research and Technology Center, Houston, Texas.

Bergmanson, J. P. G. (2000b) Endothelial complications. In *Anterior Segment Complications of Contact Lens Wear,* 2nd edn (J. A. Silbert, ed.), pp. 37–66, Butterworth-Heinemann.

Bergmanson, J. P. G. and Chu, L. W. F. (1982) Contact lens induced corneal epithelial injury. *Am. J. Optom. Physiol. Optics*, **59**, 500–506.

Bergmanson, J. P. G. and Wilson, G. S. (1989) Ultrastructural effects of sodium chloride on the corneal epithelium. *Invest. Ophthalmol. Vis. Sci.*, **30**, 116–121.

Bergmanson, J. P. G., Ruben, M. and Chu, L. W. F. (1985) Epithelial morphological response to soft hydrogel contact lenses. *Br. J. Ophthalmol.*, **69**, 373–379.

Bergmanson, J. P. G., Sheldon, T. M. and Goosey, J. D. (1999) Fuchs' endothelial dystrophy: A fresh look at an aging disease. *Ophthal. Physiol. Opt.*, **19**, 210–222.

Bourne, W. M., Hodge, D. O. and McLaren, J. W. (1999) Estimation of corneal endothelial pump function in long-term contact lens wearers. *Invest. Ophthalmol. Vis. Sci.*, **40**, 603–611.

Bozzola, J. J. and Russell, L. D. (1992) *Electron Microscopy*, Jones & Bartlett.

Bron, A. J., Tripathi, F. C. and Tripathi, B. J. (1997) Development of the human eye. In *Wolff's Anatomy of the Eye and Orbit*, 8th edn, pp. 620–664, Chapman & Hall.

Campos, M., Szerenyi, K., Lee, M. *et al.* (1994) Keratocyte loss after corneal de-epithelialization in primates and rabbits. *Arch. Ophthalmol.*, **112**, 254–260.

Carlson, K. H., Bourne, W. M. and Brubaker, R. F. (1988) Effect of long-term contact lens wear on corneal endothelial cell morphology and function. *Invest. Ophthalmol. Vis. Sci.*, **29**, 185–193.

Collin, S. P. and Collin, H. B. (2000) A comparative SEM study of the vertebrate corneal epithelium. *Cornea*, **19**, 218–230.

Cook, C. S., Ozanics, V. and Jakobiec, F. A. (1999) Prenatal development of the eye and its adnexa. In *Biomedical Foundations of Ophthalmology*, pp. 1–93, Lippincott, Williams & Wilkins.

Cotsarelis, G. C. S., Dong, G., Sun, T. T. and Lavker, R. M. (1989) Existence of slow-cycling limbal epithelial basal cells that can be preferentially stimulated to proliferate: Implications on epithelial stem cells. *Cell*, **57**, 201–209.

Dohlman, C. H., Gasset, A. R. and Rose, J. (1968) The effect of the absence of corneal epithelium or endothelium on the stromal keratocytes. *Invest. Ophthalmol. Vis. Sci.*, **7**, 520–534.

Doughty, M. J. (1989) Toward a quantitative analysis of corneal endothelial cell morphology: A review of techniques and their application. *Optom. Vis. Sci.*, **66**, 626–642.

Doughty, M. J. (1990) The ambiguous coefficient of variation: polymegethism of the corneal endothelium and central corneal thickness. *Int. Contact Lens Clin.*, **17**, 240–246.

Doughty, M. J. and Zaman, M. L. (2000) Human corneal thickness and its impact on intraocular pressure measures: A review and meta-analysis approach. *Surv. Ophthalmol.*, **44**, 367–408.

Doughty, M. J., Bergmanson, J. P. G. and Blocker, Y. (1997) Shrinkage and distortion of the rabbit corneal endothelial cell mosaic caused by a high osmolarity glutaraldehyde-formaldehyde fixative compared to glutaraldehyde. *Tissue Cell*, **29**, 533–547.

Doughty, M. J., Searbert, W., Bergmanson, J. P. G. *et al.* A quantitative transmission electron microscopy study of the keratocytes of the corneal stroma of albino rabbits. *Tissue Cell*, (in press).

Dua, H. S. and Azuara-Blanco, A. (2000) Limbal stem cells of the corneal epithelium. *Surv. Ophthalmol.*, **44**, 415–425.

Duke-Elder, S. and Wybar, K. C. (1961) Cornea. In *The Anatomy of the Visual System. System of Ophthalmology*, Vol. II (S. Duke-Elder, ed.), pp. 95–131, Henry Kimpton.

Efron, N. (1999) Corneal endothelium. In *Contact Lens Complications*, pp. 129–146, Butterworth-Heinemann.

Gillette, T. E., Chandler, J. W. and Greiner, J. V. (1982) Langerhans cells. A review of their nature with emphasis on their immunologic function. *Ophthalmology*, **89**, 700–709.

Goldman, J. N. and Benedek, G. B. (1967) The relationship between morphology and transparency in the nonswelling corneal stroma of the shark. *Invest. Ophthalmol. Vis. Sci.*, **6**, 574–580.

Hanna, C. and O'Brien, J. E. (1960) Cell production and migration in the epithelial layer of the cornea. *Arch. Ophthalmol.*, **64**, 536–541.

Hayashi, K., Sueishi, K., Tanaka, K. and Inomata, H. (1986) Immunohistochemical evidence of the origin of human corneal endothelial cells and keratocytes. *Graefe's Arch. Clin. Exp. Ophthalmol.*, **224**, 452–466.

Hayat, M. A. (1973) *Principles and Techniques of Electron Microscopy, Vol. 3: Biological Applications*, Van Nostrand Reinhold Co.

Hazlett, L. D., McClellan, S. M., Hulme, E. B. H. *et al.* (1999) Extended wear contact lens usage induces Langerhans cell migration into cornea. *Exp. Eye Res.*, **69**, 575–577.

Hill, J. C., Sarvan, J., Maske, R. and Els, W. J. (1994) Evidence that UV-B irradiation decreases corneal Langerhans cells and improves corneal graft survival in the rabbit. *Transplantation*, **57**, 1281–1284.

Hirsch, L. W., Yamauchi, K., Enger, C. *et al.* (1989) Quantitative analysis of wide-field specular microscopy. II. Precision of sampling from the central corneal endothelium. *Invest. Ophthalmol. Vis. Sci.*, **30**, 1972–1978.

Hirst, L.W., Auer, C., Cohn, J. *et al.* (1984) Specular microscopy of hard contact lens wearers. *Ophthalmology,* **91**, 1147–1153.

Holden, B. A., Sweeney, D. F., Vannas, A. *et al.* (1985) Effects of long-term extended contact lens wear on the human cornea. *Invest. Ophthalmol. Vis. Sci.,* **26**, 1489–1501.

Hornhinnans, C. F. (1857) *Histologi.* Thesis, Upsala University Medical School, Stockholm.

Johnson, D. H., Bourne, W. M. and Campbell, R. J. (1982) The ultrastructure of Descemet's membrane: I. Changes with age in normal corneas. *Arch. Ophthalmol.,* **100**, 1942–1947.

Komai, Y. and Tatsuo, U. (1991) The three dimensional organization of collagen fibrils in the human cornea and sclera. *Invest. Ophthalmol. Vis. Sci.,* **32**, 2244–2258.

Kruse, F. E. (1994) Stem cells and corneal epithelial regeneration. *Eye,* **8**, 170–183.

Krutsinger, B. D. and Bergmanson, J. P. G. (1985) Corneal epithelial response to hypotonic exposure. *Int. Eye Care,* **1**, 440–443.

Kuwabara, T. (1978) Current concepts in anatomy and histology of the cornea. *Contact Intraoc. Lens Med. J.,* **4**, 101–132.

Ladage, P. M., Yauramoto, K., Ren, D. H. *et al.* (2000) Basal epithelial cell turnover following RGP extended contact lens wear in the rabbit cornea. *Invest. Ophthalmol. Vis. Sci.,* **41**, S75.

Li, H. F., Petroll, W. M., Moller-Pedersen, T. *et al.* (1997) Epithelial and corneal thickness measurements by in vivo confocal microscopy through focusing (CMTF). *Curr. Eye Res.,* **16**, 214–221.

MacRae, S. M., Matsuda, M., Shellans, S. *et al.* (1986) The effects of hard and soft contact lenses on the corneal endothelium. *Am. J. Ophthalmol.,* **102**, 50–57.

Marshall, J. and Grindle, F. J. (1978) Fine structure of the cornea and its development. *Trans. Ophthalmol. Soc. UK,* **98**, 320–328.

McCartney, M. D. and Cantu-Crouch, D. (1992) Rabbit corneal epithelial wound repair: tight junction reformation. *Curr. Eye Res.,* **11**, 15–24.

Millodot, M. (1976a) Corneal sensitivity in people with the same and with different iris color. *Invest. Ophthalmol. Vis. Sci.,* **15**, 861–862.

Millodot, M. (1976b) Effect of the length of wear of contact lenses on corneal sensitivity. *Acta Ophthalmol.,* **54**, 721–730.

Millodot, M. and O'Leary, D. J. (1981) Corneal fragility and its relationship to sensitivity. *Acta Ophthalmol.,* **59**, 820–826

Moller-Pedersen, T. and Ehlers, N. (1995) A three-dimensional study of the human corneal keratocyte density. *Curr. Eye Res.,* **14**, 459–464.

Moller-Pedersen, T., Ledet, T. and Ehlers, N. (1994) The keratocyte density of human donor corneas. *Curr. Eye Res.,* **13**, 163–169.

Müller, L. J., Pels, L. and Vrensen, G. F. J. M. (1995) Novel aspects of the ultrastructural organization of human corneal keratocytes. *Invest. Ophthalmol. Vis. Sci.,* **36**, 2557–2567.

Müller, L. J., Pels, L. and Vrensen, G. F. J. M. (1996) Ultrastructural organization of human corneal nerves. *Invest. Ophthalmol. Vis. Sci.,* **37**, 476–488.

Petroll, W. M., Boettcher, K., Barry, P. *et al.* (1995) Quantitative assessment of antero-posterior keratocyte density in the normal rabbit cornea. *Cornea,* **14**, 3–9.

Polse, K. A., Brand, R. J. and Cohen, S. R. (1990) Hypoxic effects on corneal hydration control in Fuchs' dystrophy. *Optom. Vis. Sci.*, **68**, 831.

Pritchard, N., Jones, L., Dumbleton, K. and Fonn, D. (2000) Epithelial inclusions in association with mucin ball development in high-oxygen permeability hydrogel lenses. *Optom. Vis. Sci.*, **77**, 68–72.

Ren, D. H., Petroll, W. M., Jester, J. V. and Cavanagh, H. D. (1999) The effect of rigid gas permeable contact lens wear on proliferation of rabbit corneal and conjunctival epithelial cells. *Contact Lens Assoc. Ophthalmol. J.*, **25**, 136–141.

Schoessler, J. P. and Lowther, G. E. (1971) Slit lamp observations of corneal oedema. *Am. J. Optom. Arch. Am. Acad. Optom.*, **48**, 666–671.

Schoessler, J. P. and Woloschak, M. J. (1981) Corneal endothelium in veteran PMMA contact lens wearers. *Int. Contact Lens Clin.*, **8**, 19–26.

Thoft, R. A. and Friend, J. (1983) The X,Y,Z hypothesis of corneal epithelial maintenance. *Invest. Ophthalmol. Vis. Sci.*, **24**, 1442–1443.

Watsky, M. A. (1995) Keratocyte gap junctional communication in normal and wounded rabbit corneas and human corneas. *Invest. Ophthalmol. Vis. Sci.*, **36**, 2568–2576.

You, X. K., Bergmanson, J. P. G., Zheng, X. M. *et al.* (1995) Effect of corticosteroids on rabbit corneal keratocytes after photorefractive keratectomy. *J. Refract. Surg.*, **11**, 460–467.

Zieske, J. D. (1994) Perpetuation of stem cells in the eye. *Eye*, **8**, 163–169.

5 Corneal topography

Stephen D. Klyce

Introduction

The front surface of the cornea with its normally smooth tear film provides two-thirds of the refractive power of the eye. Disruptions in the tear film and induction of irregularity in corneal shape, which can occur as a complication of contact lens wear can, therefore, degrade the optical quality of the cornea, and reduce visual acuity. Such distortions in the corneal surface can be so subtle as to escape detection with the usual biomicroscope examination. Retinoscopy can show fairly slight distortions in the retinal image that can arise from cornea/tear film imperfections, but retinoscopy does not reveal the nature and/or locus of the aberrating medium; corneal back surface, lenticular and retinal anomalies can distort vision as well.

The development of the photokeratoscope, such as the Nidek PKS–1000 (Riss *et al.*, 1991) and the Corneascope (Rowsey *et al.*, 1981) helped diagnose mild keratoconus and manage astigmatism in corneal grafts. In 1979, refractive surgery in the form of radial keratotomy entered clinical practice in the USA, and this, along with advances in the microcomputer arena, provided the impetus and capability for the development of improved methods for analysing corneal shape.

Development of the corneal topographer

In 1981, Doss and co-workers scanned Corneascope photographs to calculate corneal powers from mire size and shape. These data were presented in the form of a numerical plot. Subsequently, Klyce (1984) demonstrated a method for reconstructing corneal shape and power by digitizing mires from Nidek photokeratoscope photographs. In this work, graphical plots using three-dimensional wire-mesh models were used to depict corneal topography, as condensing the thousands of data points collected from the photokeratoscope photographs was necessary to permit clinical utility. The final graphical presentation form of these data, which has become the international standard, was the colour-coded contour map of corneal powers developed by Maguire *et al.* (1987).

Units of measure

Corneal power or curvature had been measured clinically for nearly a century before the advent of corneal topographers. First, surface corneal curvature can be expressed directly using millimetres, which is the preferred unit for contact lens practitioners. However, for the purpose of evaluating the optics of the eye and refractive errors, the most convenient unit is the 'dioptre'. The relationship between the two is provided by the 'keratometric index' (0.3375) such that 'mm' can be converted to 'dioptres' and vice versa simply by dividing the measured amount into 0.3375. The dioptric power so obtained is the power of the whole cornea (front surface approximately 48 D less back surface approximately 5 D); however, the above relationship fails to accurately predict corneal power changes, particularly when only the anterior surface curvature is modified as with refractive surgery (Swinger and Barker, 1984; Arffa *et al.*, 1986). Nevertheless, for consistency of clinical interpretation, the 'keratometric index' has been carried over for the expression of corneal power in corneal topographers. On the average, normal adult human corneal power is about 43 D with this convention. For the 43 D cornea, anterior surface curvature is thus 7.85 mm (i.e. 337.5 divided by 43).

The colour-coded map

The colour-coded contour map of corneal powers conveys topographic information with the concept of colour association and pattern recognition. A colour spectrum was chosen so that powers near the norm were shown as green, powers lower than this were shown as cool colours, and high corneal powers were shown as warm colours. Only a few distinct, recognizable colours were chosen over the central range of corneal powers so that a specific power interval could be easily identified. The contours in these maps provide for pattern recognition, including the identification of naturally occurring topographies such as corneal cylinder ('bow tie' pattern), keratoconus (local area of steepening), and pellucid marginal degeneration (inferior arcuate steepening), as well as features associated with refractive surgery, such as optical zone size, centration and central islands.

Standardized scales

The utility of corneal topography can be influenced by the colour spectrum and contour interval implemented. The colours and dioptric interval originally proposed (Maguire *et al.*, 1987) have been modified in a number of ways by manufacturers, and efforts to standardize corneal topography have not been successful. Following the work of Maguire *et al.* (1987), Wilson and co-workers (Wilson *et al.*, 1993) introduced a more practical scale (the 'Klyce–Wilson scale'), which ranged from 28.0 to 65.5 dioptres in equal 1.5 dioptre intervals. Although the 1.5 dioptre interval may not be sensitive enough for topographers with broad mires and less spatial resolution, it was found to be adequate for normal clinical use.

The diagnostic adequacy of the Klyce–Wilson scale was evaluated in a clinical series that included normal corneas, contact lens-wearing corneas, early to moderate and advanced keratoconus, penetrating keratoplasties, extracapsular cataract surgery, excimer laser photorefractive keratectomy, radial keratotomy, aphakic epikeratoplasty and myopic epikeratoplasty. It was found that the correct interpretation for all cases could be made with the 1.5 dioptre scale without resorting to a 1.0 dioptre or lower interval scale (Wilson *et al.*, 1993). Additionally, the 1.5 dioptre scale proved to be broad enough to cover the full range of powers encountered in the study. The routine use of a fixed standard scale showing only adequate detail and not redundant information or extraneous measurement noise is essential for efficient and accurate clinical interpretation.

Although it has been traditional that corneal topographers offer adaptable scales that are self-adjusting to the range of powers found for a given cornea, their use can be misleading. Such scales can make grossly irregular corneas look uncomplicated and normal corneas look complex, with extensive amounts of irregular astigmatism. Such adaptive scales should be avoided except as an adjunct to examine details of corneal topography.

Corneal topographers

There is a constantly growing number of devices for automatically measuring corneal topography, and a variety of optical principles have been adopted. These are outlined below.

Placido disc

The Corneal Modelling System (CMS; Computed Anatomy, New York, USA) was the first of a growing number of devices for automatically measuring corneal topography and used the videocapture of Placido disc images to do so. The Placido disc approach has been the most prevalent of the methods (Table 5.1). Some of these have been validated in terms of accuracy and reproducibility as there can be considerable differences in the results obtained with the various machines (Hannush *et al.*, 1989; Wilson *et al.*, 1992; Belin and Zloty, 1993; Legeais *et al.*, 1993; Maguire *et al.*, 1993; Roberts, 1994; Douthwaite, 1995; Zadnik *et al.*, 1995). Two types of Placido targets have been used. A large diameter target can be less sensitive to misalignment due to a long working distance, but is subject

Table 5.1 Corneal topographers

Manufacturer	Model(s)	Method
Alcon Surgical	EyeMap EH-290	Placido
Alliance Medical Mkts	Keratron CT; Scout	Placido
B & L Surgical	Orbscan II	Scanned slits and Placido
B & L Surgical	Orbshot	Placido
Dicon	CT-200	Placido
Euclid Systems	ET-800	Fluorescein profilometry
EyeSys/Premier	EyeSys 2000; Vista	Placido
Eyetek	CT2000	Placido
Humphrey Instruments	Atlas 991, 992	Placido
Kera Metrics	CLAS-1000	Laser holography
Medmont	E300	Placido
Oculus	Keratograph	Placido
PAR Vision Systems	CTS, Accugrid	Fluorescein profilometry
PAR Vision Systems	Intraop. CTS	Fluorescein profilometry
Sun Contact Lens Co.	SK-2000	Placido
TechnoMed Technology	C-SCAN	Placido
Tomey Technology	AutoTopographer	Placido
Topcon America Corp.	CM-1000	Placido

to data loss due to eclipse of the mires by the brow and nose of the patient. A small diameter cone-shaped target does not suffer from peripheral data loss due to shadows, but given their short working distances, these rely on automatic alignment and focus or compensation for misalignment in order to accord good accuracy.

Rasterstereography

A second technology developed to measure corneal shape is the technique of rasterstereography (Warnicki *et al.*, 1988; Arffa *et al.*, 1989;

Naufal *et al.*, 1997). With this approach, fluorescein is first instilled in the tear film, and a grid or raster pattern is projected with cobalt blue light onto the anterior surface of the eye. Images are then captured simultaneously from two directions and processed using triangulation methodology to reconstruct the shape of the cornea. This seems to be less sensitive than Placido disc topography, and this limitation along with the inconvenience of having to instil fluorescein reduces its usefulness. On the plus side, rasterstereography can measure actual corneal shape directly and without the successive approximation method used with Placido disc machines.

Scanning slit technology

The use of scanning slit beam technology can provide the opportunity to analyse both the anterior and posterior surfaces of the cornea, and was first introduced in the Corneal Modelling System by Computed Anatomy (New York, USA). Since both of these refracting surfaces, as well as corneal thickness, come into play when calculating total corneal power, measuring the position of the surfaces directly would provide an advantage. As with rasterstereography, direct measurement eliminates the potential for elevation or shape measurement errors. Further, the ability to measure corneal thickness over a broad area would provide valuable guidance to the refractive surgeon, particularly if the sensitivity were great enough to detect the local stromal thinning associated with clinical keratoconus or the kerectasia that is claimed to result when too thin a corneal stromal bed is left after a laser *in situ* keratomileusis (LASIK) procedure is performed (Seiler and Quurke, 1998).

The scanning slit technique is currently used by the Orbscan II (Bausch & Lomb, Rochester, New York, USA; Table 5.1), which employs a Placido disc for a traditional measurement of corneal anterior surface topography and a scanning slit to obtain 40 slit sections of the cornea. These images, captured in something over one second, are registered with one another and are used to reconstruct the full-thickness cornea. Subsequently, thickness profiles, surface elevation maps, and conventional topography maps are calculated and displayed.

The accuracy of the scanning slit method for measuring corneal thickness has been questioned, showing a need for independent validation studies (Yaylali *et al.*, 1997; Lattimore *et al.*, 1999). Further, the validity of scanning slit studies reporting kerectasia after LASIK has been challenged on mathematical grounds (Maloney, 1999). There could be shortcomings to the scanning slit approach that are difficult to overcome. Because the cornea is in constant motion from fixation drift, muscle tremor, pulse and nystagmus, correlated measurements must be captured simultaneously or in a minimum time period of 30 ms or less. Having a scanning slit device capturing successive slit images over a long period of time without image tracking or adequate post-capture image registration invites significant movement artefact.

Interferometry

Potentially the most accurate methodology that has been proposed to measure corneal shape is interferometry (Rottenkolber and Podbielska, 1996). Interference techniques are used in the optical industry to detect lens and mirror aberrations of subwavelength dimensions. In essence, a reference surface (or its hologram) is compared to the measured surface (cornea) and interference fringes are produced as a result of differences between the two shapes. With respect to the measurement of corneal shape, there is such a wide variation in the shapes of corneas, even among those that are normal, that it is difficult for a single interference device to represent all the variations. Examples of interference devices include a phase-modulated laser holography-based device (Shack *et al.*, 1979; Burris *et al.*, 1993) (Table 5.1) and an acoustic holographic technique (Smolek, 1994). Neither approach has yet led to a clinically accepted diagnostic tool.

Corneal topographic indexes

While the colour-coded map provides a rapid method for clinical diagnosis and is constructed from quantitative measurements taken from the corneal surface, such maps do not by themselves provide numerical values that can be used for clinical management. These might be divided into basic traditional measures used for contact lens fitting (e.g. keratometry values), indexes that could be used to assess the optical quality of the corneal surface, indexes for detecting keratoconus and, finally, indexes that could be used in artificial intelligence systems to aid in the diagnosis of corneal shape anomalies. A number of numerical systems have been developed to this end; those developed by the author and his colleagues are discussed here. The reader is referred to the Holladay Diagnostic Summary (Holladay, 1997) for an alternative system.

Basic topography indexes

Basic indexes are akin to traditional measures that are used, say, for contact lens fitting and would be intuitively familiar to clinicians.

SimK

SimK values provide the powers and axes of the steepest and flattest meridians (SimK1 and SimK2, respectively), to simulate the values provided by the keratometer (Dingeldein *et al.*, 1989). Cylinder is provided as the simple difference between SimK1 and SimK2. SimK values are calculated from mires that approximately correspond to the position on the cornea at which keratometer measurements would be obtained. SimK values correlate well with keratometry values and all corneal topographers provide this measurement. Used for fitting contact lenses and refractive surgery calculations, SimK values can be extremely valuable as a starting point for determining the quantity and axis of astigmatism during refractions in eyes with irregular corneal shapes.

Corneal eccentricity index

The 'corneal eccentricity index' (CEI) is a quantitative descriptor that indicates the eccentricity of the central cornea (Maeda *et al.*, 1994a). The CEI is generally calculated by fitting an ellipse to corneal elevation data obtained with the corneal topographer. In a study of 22 control corneas, the CEI was reported to be 0.33 ± 0.26 (mean ± 1 standard deviation), which corresponds with the prolate shape of the normal central cornea. This value is useful in contact lens fitting and for differentiating between normal prolate corneas and oblate corneas flattened by myopic refractive surgery.

Average corneal power

The 'average corneal power' (ACP) is an area-corrected average of the corneal power ahead of the entrance pupil (Maeda *et al.*, 1997). It is generally equal to the keratometric spherical equivalent except for decentred refractive surgical procedures. In such cases, ACP may be helpful to determine the average central corneal curvature for intraocular lens power calculations.

Topographic indexes and methods for measuring corneal optical quality

The development of corneal topography analysis was spurred on by the advent of refractive surgery in the late 1970s as clues were sought to complications that could arise from the induction of irregular astigmatism. This led to the development of the following, more sophisticated approaches.

Surface regularity index

The first topographic index that measured irregular astigmatism was the 'surface regularity index' (SRI) (Wilson and Klyce, 1991). The SRI measures the meridional mire to mire changes in power for the cornea over the apparent entrance pupil of the eye. These changes are summed up to provide the index, SRI. This index was correlated to the visual acuity of the eyes of a group of normal subjects as well as patients with keratoconus and corneal transplants. With this correlation, the 'potential visual acuity' (PVA) of the eye can be predicted in terms of Snellen lines.

A different approach to measuring corneal surface distortion was taken by Maloney *et al.* (1993) and Holladay (1997), who chose to find the best-fitting ellipsoid to the central cornea and then calculate the difference between this semi-ideal surface and the corneal elevation. Using clinical correlations, Holladay (1997) presents these distortions in the form of a colour-coded map of predicted regional Snellen acuity as a measure of optical quality.

Fourier methods

Fourier series are particularly good at fitting periodic functions and decomposing these into their underlying components through a transform from the spatial domain to the frequency domain. This transformation can provide average corneal power, amount and axis of regular astigmatism, and terms that can be summed to give an estimate of irregular astigmatism as well (Hjortdal *et al.*, 1995; Olsen *et al.*, 1996; Oshika *et al.*, 1998b). This approach has been used to evaluate both regular and irregular corneal astigmatism.

Ray tracing

While the SRI is a primitive form of ray tracing, a potentially more precise and sophisticated approach has been taken by several groups. Using ray tracing techniques, effective spherical aberration was found to be highly correlated with best corrected acuity in patients who had undergone photorefractive keratectomy (Seiler *et al.*, 1993). The TechnoMed C-SCAN (Table 5.1) uses ray tracing through a Gullstrand model eye to estimate visual acuity from the minimum resolvable variable. Camp *et al.* (1990) and Maguire *et al.* (1991) demonstrated a subjective ray tracing approach by calculating images that would be formed through individual corneas with irregular astigmatism.

Aberration structures

Optical systems have traditionally been studied by evaluating wavefronts, the term used to describe the optical path length of light rays through a lens system. If the optical path lengths were uniform over the pupil of the eye, there would be no aberration of the wavefront and presumably the sharpest vision could then be obtained; this would only be limited by receptor diameter and spacing in the fovea and diffraction.

Since the cornea/tear film is the major refracting interface in the eye, and since it is easily accessible, the measurement of the aberrations of the eye stemming from corneal shape imperfections has received a good deal of attention. Wavefront analysis has been applied to examine the aberration structure of the cornea before and after refractive surgery with the aim of understanding the impact on visual function (Applegate *et al.*, 1994; Applegate and Howland, 1997; Martinez *et al.*, 1998). Corneal topography data ordinarily comprise three-dimensional elements that include position on the corneal surface and dioptric power. To determine the aberration structure of a cornea, the elevations of the presurgical cornea over a specified diameter centred over the pupil are matched with the best-fitting sphere. The differences between the postoperative corneal elevations and this best-fitting sphere are found; this is called the remainder lens. This structure is then fitted with a three-dimensional Taylor polynomial equation and transformed to a Zernike polynomial series in order to examine tilt, defocus, cylinder, coma-like aberrations, spherical-like aberrations and irregular (higher order) aberrations. Analyses are performed to compare preoperative corneal aberrations with the same types of aberrations after surgery.

With this approach one can examine the aberrations for various pupil diameters generally, with a 3 mm pupil to examine daylight vision, and with a 7 mm pupil to evaluate night vision. It was found that refractive surgery –radial keratotomy (RK), photorefractive keratectomy (PRK) and laser-assisted keratomileusis (LASIK) – increases the total corneal aberrations with a 7 mm pupil. This is not surprising since the planned optical zone of these procedures typically varied from under 5 mm to 6 mm at the most. Scanning lasers, however, can be set to a 7 mm optical zone for lower refractive corrections, and in these cases total aberrations are decreased. When 3 mm pupils were assessed, the amount of induced optical aberrations was considerably less (300 times) than for the 7 mm pupil. Although coma increased slightly with the 3 mm pupil, spherical-like aberrations were actually diminished (Martinez *et al.*, 1998). More recent studies with a third-generation scanning laser (Model EC–5000, NIDEK, Gamagori, Japan) found a statistically significant decrease in total aberrations for the 3 mm pupil, providing a strong indication that refractive surgical procedures are improving significantly.

Indexes for keratoconus detection

With the high sensitivity to detect shape anomalies, corneal topographers can provide a more dependable method than retinoscopy for the detection of corneal asymmetry – the hallmark of mild keratoconus. Typically we denote keratoconus-suspect corneas as those with a small amount of localized steepening on corneal topography (Figure 5.1) with none of the other traditional clinical signs (thinning, striae, etc.). When these signs are evident, the diagnosis of clinical keratoconus is made. The

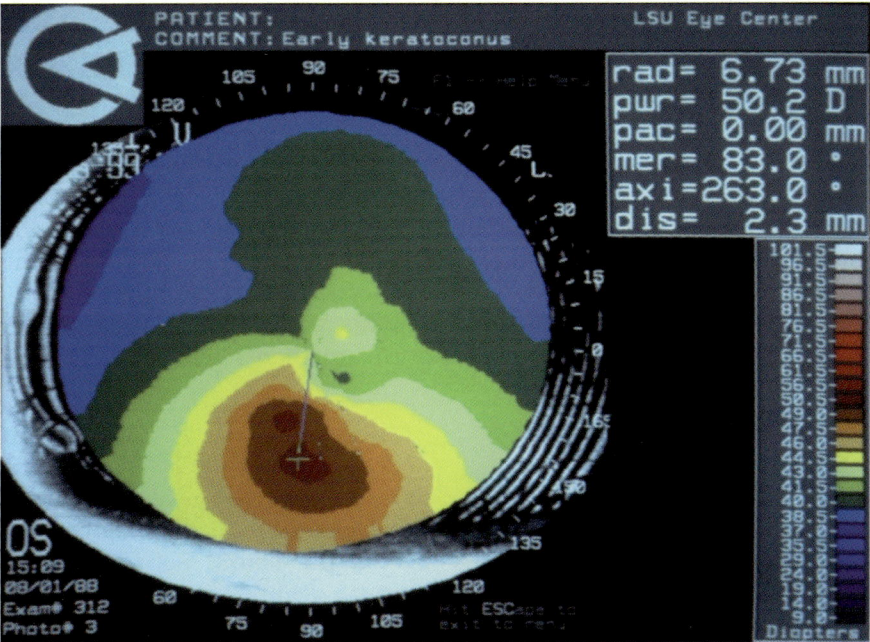

Figure 5.1 Topographic example of early keratoconus

challenge has been to establish 'cutoff' values derived from corneal topography to help make the distinction between keratoconus suspect and clinical keratoconus. Indexes derived from corneal topography have been developed to do this.

Rabinowitz and McDonnell (1989) developed algorithms for the detection of keratoconus that are available on some corneal topographers. This method uses three observations:

1. Power differences are commonly noted between the superior and inferior paracentral corneal regions in keratoconus, and this is measured as the I-S value.

2. Central corneal power (MaxK) is higher in keratoconus than normals.
3. There is commonly a difference in progression of corneal steepening in the two eyes of a keratoconus patient.

The method yields a positive result for a keratoconus suspect (KCS) if the central corneal power is greater than 47.2 D. It also yields a positive result for a KCS if the I-S value is greater than 1.4 D. The method yields a positive result for clinical keratoconus (KC) if the central corneal power is greater than 48.7 D or if the I-S value is greater than 1.9 D.

An expert system was developed by Maeda and co-workers (Maeda *et al.*, 1994b, 1995a) to extend this approach to autodiagnosis. With this method, discriminant analysis is used to produce the 'keratoconus prediction index' (KPI). The KPI is obtained from topographic indexes designed to capture the characteristics seen in keratoconus maps of local abnormal elevations in corneal power. These include the 'differential sector index' (DSI), 'opposite sector index' (OSI), and 'centre/surround index' (CSI). Several other indexes were used as well to increase the specificity of the method: the 'surface asymmetry index' (SAI), the 'irregular astigmatism index' (IAI), and the 'per cent area analysed' (AA). The output of the discriminant analyser was fed to a binary decision tree to further enhance the performance of this method.

Indexes for neural networks

A more sophisticated approach for classification of corneal topography and detection of topographic abnormalities than that developed by Maeda and co-workers (1994b, 1995a) is the neural network model involving artificial intelligence (Maeda *et al.*, 1995b). This method entails automated pattern interpretation through the training of a neural network computer program. Smolek and Klyce (1997) extended this approach by producing a method that obtained 100% accuracy, specificity and sensitivity in both the training set as well as, importantly, a test set to which the neural network was naïve.

Key clinical applications

An important application of corneal topography, already discussed above, is the detection of corneal abnormalities that may be hereditary (e.g. keratoconus), iatrogenic (e.g. post-keratoplasty) or due to disease (e.g. corneal ectasia). Two further key applications of this technology are contact lens wear and refractive surgery.

Contact lens wear

By virtue of the physical apposition of the contact lens and cornea, physical forces can act to change the shape of both the lens and the eye. Indeed, both types of change have been documented and both can have important clinical sequelae. Videokeratoscopy allows various indexes of corneal shape change to be measured so that the effects of various lens types and wearing modalities can be evaluated.

Conventional lens fitting

Ruiz-Montenegro et al. (1993) reported SAI mean values (± standard error of mean) associated with the following forms of lens wear: non-lens wearing controls, 0.35 ± 0.03; PMMA, 0.86 ± 0.22; daily wear RGP, 0.48 ± 0.09; daily wear soft, 0.48 ± 0.11; extended wear soft, 0.46 ± 0.08. The SAI was statistically significantly greater than the control group for all forms of lens wear except for the category 'daily wear soft'.

The clinical significance of this finding was highlighted by the fact that the authors observed a correlation between the nature of corneal deformation and the fit of the lens. For example, a superior riding rigid lens was associated with superior flattening, thus explaining the increase in SAI in that case. Such correlations were only observed in PMMA and RGP lens wearers, and an example is depicted in Figures 5.2 and 5.3.

Ruiz-Montenegro et al. (1993) also reported SRI mean values (± standard error of mean) associated with the same lens-wearing groups: non-lens-wearing controls, 0.41 ± 0.04; PMMA, 1.17 ± 0.34; daily wear RGP, 0.93 ± 0.18; daily wear soft, 0.52 ± 0.08; extended wear soft, 0.51 ± 0.06. The SRI was statistically significantly greater than the control group for PMMA and daily RGP lens wear but not for daily or extended soft lens wear. The authors observed an association in PMMA and RGP lens wearers whereby a decrease in best spectacle-corrected visual acuity occurred in patients displaying an increased SRI. The patients did not suffer significant discomfort.

The precise pathological processes that explain corneal shape changes characterized by SAI and SRI are difficult to derive because research has not been conducted to differentiate mechanisms that underlie changes in corneal symmetry and regularity. In the absence of other explanatory mechanisms, one can only conclude that surface asymmetry and irregularity are caused by differing contributions of two key factors – physical pressure by the contact lens and eyelids, and lens-induced hypoxia.

It may also be true that individual differences in corneal rigidity may be a governing factor. Ruiz-Montenegro et al. (1993) noted that much of the variance in their data could be attributed to a small number of

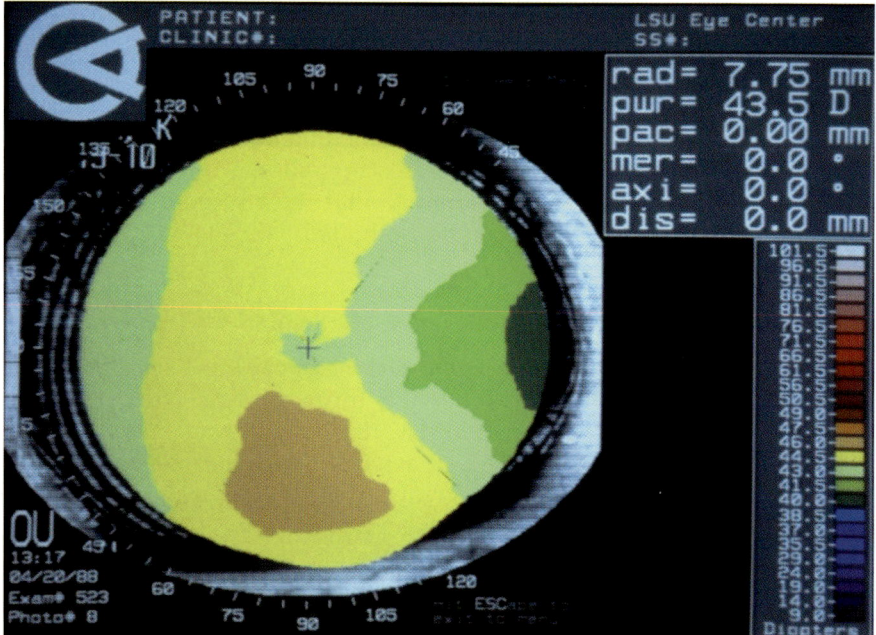

Figure 5.2 Topographic map of cornea immediately following removal of a high-riding PMMA lens. Note superior corneal flattening

patients displaying large alterations in SAI and SRI. The implication here is that some patients with 'softer' or more pliable corneas will be more susceptible to lens-induced shape changes, and that such patients will be slower to recover.

Orthokeratology

Refractive correction with contact lenses has been a long-standing goal of clinicians. Initial carefully controlled studies showed that the results were unpredictable and not long lasting. In fact, without a careful fitting plan, we are aware that visually significant and apparently permanent contact lens moulding can have a serious negative impact on the optical quality of the cornea. However, recent advances in lens design, in particular the reverse geometry lenses, have breathed new life into the approach. Nichols and co-workers (Nichols *et al.*, 2000) report significant topographic effects including corneal flattening and a reduction in shape factor due to a central corneal thinning after a regimen of overnight wear of RGP reverse geometry lenses. This is presented as a means of temporarily reducing myopia that was sustained over an 8-hour period of

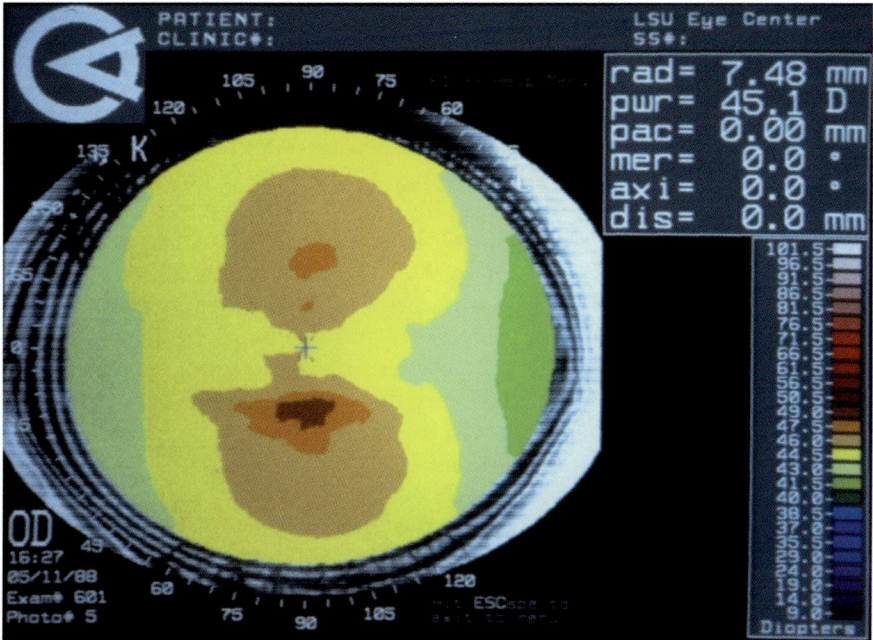

Figure 5.3 Topographic map of same cornea depicted in Figure 5.2, 3 weeks following lens removal. The cornea has recovered normal with-the-rule astigmatism

non-wear. The apparent rapidity of central corneal flattening after just one night of wear of this type of lens is striking. The authors of the study suggest that the flattening is primarily due to a redistribution of the corneal epithelium toward the corneal periphery. Efron (2000) has recently challenged the findings of Nichols *et al.* (2000), citing problems with their experimental methodology.

Refractive surgery

The development of sensitive and reliable methods for the detection of keratoconus, such as those noted above, underscore the importance of corneal topographers in refractive surgery. It is now the standard of care to routinely screen patients with corneal topography prior to refractive surgery. This is particularly important since patients with corneal topographical abnormalities are often not tolerant of spectacles or contact lenses. A disproportionate number of these patients seek out refractive surgery as an alternative, but in most cases this alternative is not recommended.

Topographic screening prior to refractive surgery is also essential for the patient with any history of contact lens wear. Typically, patients are asked to discontinue contact lens wear two weeks prior to an evaluation for suitability to be subjected to a refractive procedure. This may not be an adequate time period to allow a cornea to relax to a stable shape if there has been contact lens moulding. While soft contact lenses may produce less potential for moulding than rigid contact lenses, the average time to achieve corneal stability after symptomatic contact lens wear can be several months (Wilson *et al.*, 1990). Therefore, the general recommendation for topographic screening prior to refractive surgery is for the contact lens patient to discontinue wear and to have repeat topography examinations performed every 2–3 weeks until the topography and/or the refraction is stable. For a 3.00 D myope who has 1.00 D of contact lens moulding, the wait for stability will mean the difference between a good result and a poor or unstable outcome.

Corneal topography has also been extremely useful for the evaluation of those patients who are symptomatic after surgery. The symptoms of distortion, halos, glare and monocular diplopia are often found to be caused by a small or decentred optical zone, central islands, or unclassifiable irregular astigmatism. With some of these cases, custom-designed laser treatments may be the best alternative to restoration of functional vision. Reverse geometry contact lenses have also received some success in masking irregular astigmatism after refractive surgery, to the chagrin of the refractive surgeon and the frustration of the patient.

Radial keratotomy

Topographic examples of some of these refractive surgeries for the correction of myopia are instructive because they can illustrate some of the complications that may arise. Radial keratotomy (RK), which began the refractive surgery revolution in the early 1980s, was successful in a large number of patients. By far the most common complication was the lack of precision in the outcome due to inability to fine-tune the procedure. The worst optical complication resulted from micro- and macroperforations where the diamond knife penetrated into the anterior chamber. This usually resulted in long-standing irregular astigmatism (Figure 5.4).

Photorefractive keratectomy

With the adaptation of the 193 nm excimer laser to stromal tissue sculpting, came photorefractive keratectomy (PRK). Originally, these procedures were performed with beams that were several millimetres wide, and whose ablation area was controlled with an expanding or

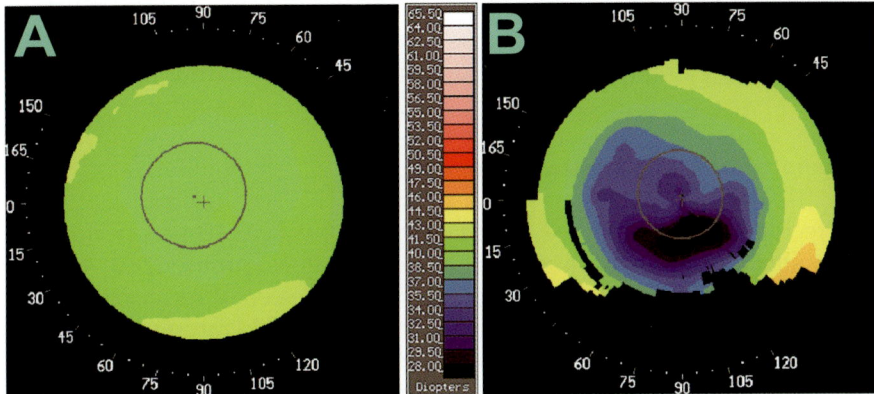

Figure 5.4 Topographic examples of radial keratotomy (RK). (A) Excellent result with a uniform, lowered central corneal power. (B) Pronounced irregular astigmatism remains 11 years after eventful radial keratotomy in which the diamond blade penetrated too deeply and entered the anterior chamber

contracting iris diaphragm. Several technical limitations of the procedure produced irregular astigmatism in a fraction of the cases. Some of these were due to the laser optics becoming degraded by the high-energy ultraviolet light. By far the most troubling form of irregular astigmatism was the central island – a central area of poorly ablated stroma (Figure 5.5). A number of hypotheses have been presented to explain this feature

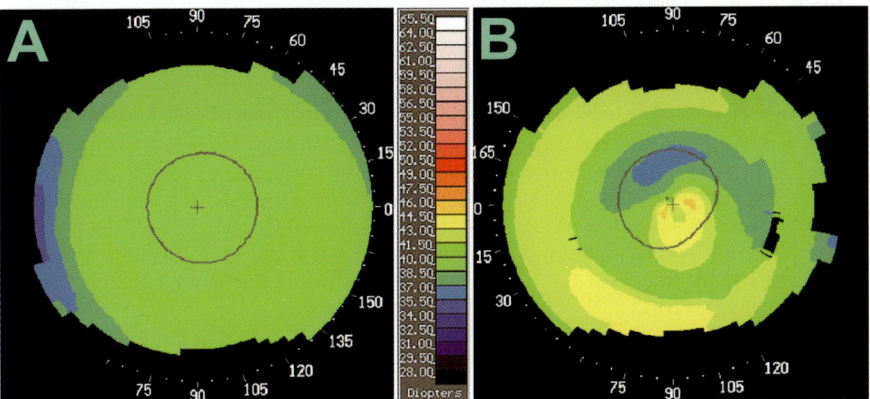

Figure 5.5 Topographic examples of photorefractive keratectomy (PRK) with the excimer laser. (A) Good result in a low myope. (B) A large central island/peninsula of less treated cornea is prominent in this case. This form of irregular astigmatism was prevalent with early model area ablating excimer lasers, but does not occur with the later model small spot scanning excimer lasers

(Oshika *et al.*, 1998a), and its effects on vision can be symptomatic. With the development of scanning lasers, central islands are no longer a problem as they seem to be related entirely to the ablating method.

Automated lamellar keratectomy

The technique of automated lamellar keratectomy (ALK) was performed for a short period of time after microkeratomes proliferated. In this procedure, a cap of stroma is sectioned off and a second refractive lenslet of tissue removed with a second pass of the microkeratome. The major problem with this procedure was unclassifiable irregular astigmatism due to irregularities in the blades, and microstriae from poor apposition of the cap on the stromal bed. Examples of topographic outcomes obtained with this procedure are shown in Figure 5.6.

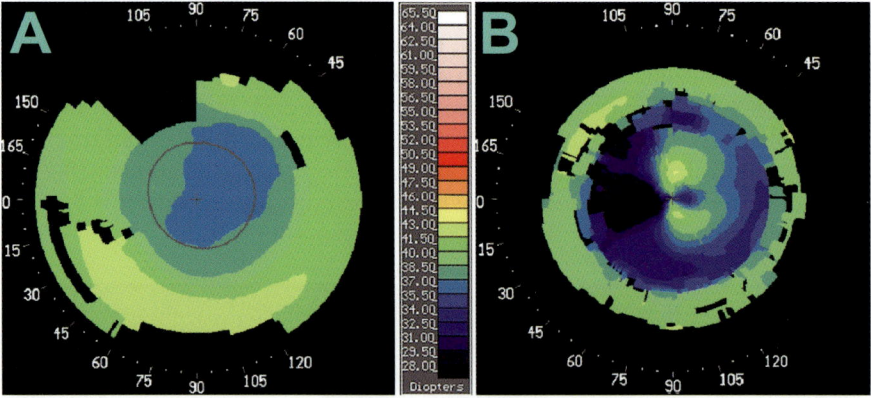

Figure 5.6 Topographic examples of automated lamellar keratectomy (ALK). In this refractive surgical procedure, a microkeratome is used to remove an anterior cap or stroma and then to make a second refractive cut removing a lenticule of stromal tissue. (A) Excellent result after ALK. (B) Severe irregular astigmatism can result with ALK because of microstriations and chatter marks produced by the microkeratome. This procedure is not currently recommended for practice

Laser in situ keratomileusis

Whereas ALK failed in its acceptance, it was adapted to laser *in situ* keratomileusis (LASIK) wherein a stromal cap (with a hinge) is made with a microkeratome, and the refractive lenslet is removed in a carefully controlled fashion with an excimer laser. The ablation made by the laser is generally a spherical correction; if there are chatter marks on the stromal bed from the microkeratome, these are preserved and simply moved deeper into the tissue. Microstriae and occasional central islands can still result; however, if the cap is repositioned on the stromal bed carefully and fully aligned with its original position, then the microkeratome chatter marks from the blade fit back together and do not cause irregular astigmatism. An example of a good result and a complication are shown in Figure 5.7.

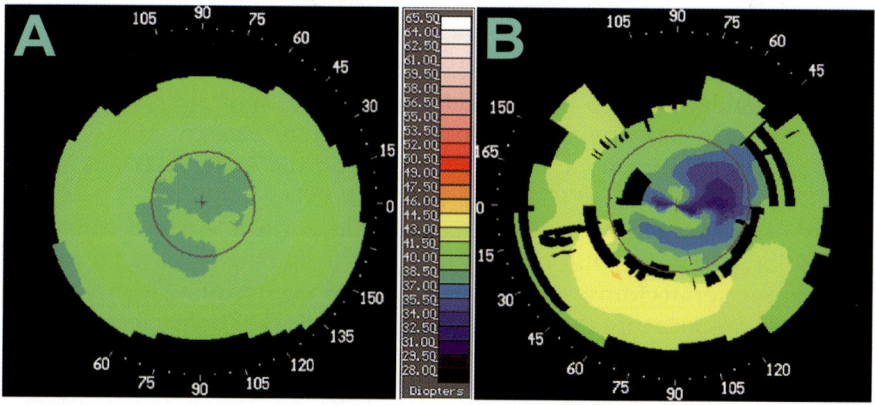

Figure 5.7 Topographic examples after laser *in situ* keratomileusis (LASIK). In this procedure, a microkeratome is used to make an anterior stroma cut to produce a cap of stroma connected to the stromal bed by a hinge of tissue. The cap is then reflected back, and the excimer laser is used to make the refractive element. The cap is then placed back on the stromal bed. Any chatter marks made during the microkeratome pass are not removed by the laser, but rather are displaced posteriorly. Hence, when the cap is replaced, the irregularities are normally aligned, limiting induced irregular astigmatism. (A) An excellent LASIK result, well-centred and uniform. (B) A high amount of irregular astigmatism present after LASIK and poor cap alignment

Conclusions

What can we expect in the future? Corneal topography has come a long way in the 15 years since the first commercial device was introduced. While companies that manufacture corneal topographers are refining their products by adding artificial intelligence, improving contact lens applications and introducing low-cost and hand-held devices, we appear to be on the brink of a revolution. There has been an enormous resurgence of interest in an old technology used to perfect the optics of microscopes and telescopes – spatially resolved refractometry – which was first introduced to ophthalmology a decade ago (Penney *et al.*, 1993).

As discussed above, determination of the aberration structure of the cornea from topography data can help in understanding the optical quality of the corneal surface after refractive surgery. However, although keratorefractive surgery is performed on the corneal surface (PRK) and within the cornea (LASIK) to correct ametropias, the goal of the procedure should be to correct the refractive error of the whole eye. Most refractive surgical procedures correct vision just as spectacles do with an attempted sphero-cylindrical change. However, as excimer lasers become more sophisticated, it is becoming possible to make complex shape changes on the corneal surface. Examples of such commercial products include the 'custom cornea' feature of the Summit/Autonomous Technologies (Orlando, Florida, USA) LadarVision flying spot excimer laser, the VISX excimer laser with its 'custom ablation pattern' (CAP; VISX Corporation, Sunnyvale, California, USA), and the ARK–10000/EC–5000 from Nidek Corporation (Gamagori, Japan).

With the capability to custom carve the corneal surface came the realization that correcting corneal irregular astigmatism, as with photo-therapeutic keratectomy, was a good first step to improving visual acuity. But if one can measure the optical aberrations of the whole eye on a point by point basis, then one might be able to use a scanning laser to modify the cornea to correct total optical aberrations. As a result, a number of aberrometers have been developed specifically for ophthalmic use, and these wavefront sensors are becoming the front ends to excimer lasers used in refractive surgery. Coupled with the data available from corneal topography, these wavefront sensors hold tremendous promise. However, the main limiting factor with the technology seems to be that of alignment. One must measure the ocular wavefront and the corneal topography, align these two data sets, and then align the resulting calculated treatment on the cornea during surgery. This is no simple task, and eye tracking of the dilated pupil margins is probably not going to be adequate to the task. Nevertheless, this is a new exciting frontier in refractive correction, and the potential advantages to vision science and our patients may well be considerable.

Acknowledgements

This work was supported in part by USA Public Health Service grants EY03311 and EY02377 from the National Eye Institute, National Institutes of Health, Bethesda, Maryland, USA. Professor Klyce has no financial interest in the subject matter of this chapter at this time.

References

Applegate, R. A. and Howland, H. C. (1997) Refractive surgery, optical aberrations, and visual performance. *J. Refract. Corneal Surg.*, **13**, 295–299.

Applegate, R. A., Howland, H. C., Buettner, L. *et al.* (1994) Changes in the aberration structure of the RK cornea from videokeratographic measurements. *Invest. Ophthalmol. Vis. Sci. (Suppl.)*, **35**, 1740.

Arffa, R. C., Klyce, S. D. and Busin, M. (1986) Keratometry in epikeratophakia. *J. Refract. Corneal Surg.*, **2**, 61–64.

Arffa, R. C., Warnicki, J. W. and Rehkopf, P. G. (1989) Corneal topography using rasterstereography. *J. Refract. Corneal Surg.*, **5**, 414–417.

Belin, M. W. and Zloty, P. (1993) Accuracy of the PAR corneal topography system with spatial misalignment. *Contact Lens Assoc. Ophthalmol. J.*, **19**, 64–68.

Burris, T. E., Baker, P. C., Ayer, C. T. *et al.* (1993) Flattening of central corneal curvature with intrastromal corneal rings of increasing thickness: an eye-bank eye study. *J. Cataract Refract. Surg. (Suppl.)*, **19**, 182–187.

Camp, J. J., Maguire, L. J., Cameron, B. M. and Robb, R. A. (1990) A computer model for the evaluation of the effect of corneal topography on optical performance. *Am. J. Ophthalmol.*, **109**, 379–386.

Dingeldein, S. A., Klyce, S. D. and Wilson, S. E. (1989) Quantitative descriptors of corneal shape derived from computer-assisted analysis of photokeratographs. *J. Refract. Corneal Surg.*, **5**, 372–378.

Doss, J. D., Hutson, R. L., Rowsey, J. J. and Brown, R. (1981) Method for calculation of corneal profile and power distribution. *Arch. Ophthalmol.*, **99**, 1261–1265.

Douthwaite, W. A. (1995) EyeSys corneal topography measurement applied to calibrated ellipsoidal convex surfaces. *Br. J. Ophthalmol.*, **79**, 797–801.

Efron, N. (2000) Overnight orthokeratology (correspondence). *Optom. Vis. Sci.*, **77**, 627–629.

Hannush, S. B., Crawford, S. L., Waring, G. O. *et al.* (1989) Accuracy and precision of keratometry, photokeratoscopy, and corneal modeling on calibrated steel balls. *Arch. Ophthalmol.*, **107**, 1235–1239.

Hjortdal, J. O., Erdmann, L. and Bek, T. (1995) Fourier analysis of video-keratographic data. A tool for separation of spherical, regular astigmatic and irregular astigmatic corneal power components. *Ophthal. Physiol. Opt.*, **15**, 171–185.

Holladay, J. T. (1997) Corneal topography using the Holladay Diagnostic Summary. *J. Cataract Refract. Surg.*, **23**, 209–221.

Klyce, S. D. (1984) Computer-assisted corneal topography: high resolution graphical presentation and analysis of keratoscopy. *Invest. Ophthalmol. Vis. Sci.*, **25**, 1426–1435.

Lattimore, M. R. Jr, Kaupp, S., Schallhorn, S. and Lewis, R. (1999) Orbscan pachymetry: implications of repeated measures and diurnal variation analysis. *Ophthalmology*, **106**, 977–981.

Legeais, J. M., Ren, Q., Simon, G. and Parel, J. M. (1993) Computer-assisted corneal topography: accuracy and reproducibility of the topographic modeling system. *J. Refract. Corneal Surg.*, **9**, 347–357.

Maeda, N., Klyce, S. D., Hamano, H. (1994a) Alteration of corneal asphericity in rigid gas permeable contact lens induced warpage. *Contact Lens Assoc. Ophthalmol. J.*, **20**, 27–31.

Maeda, N., Klyce, S. D., Smolek, M. K. and Thompson, H. W. (1994b) Automated keratoconus screening with corneal topography analysis. *Invest. Ophthalmol. Vis. Sci.*, **35**, 2749–2757.

Maeda, N., Klyce, S. D. and Smolek, M. K. (1995a) Comparison of methods for detecting keratoconus using videokeratography. *Arch. Ophthalmol.*, **113**, 870–874.

Maeda, N., Klyce, S. D. and Smolek, M. K. (1995b) Neural network classification of corneal topography. Preliminary demonstration. *Invest. Ophthalmol. Vis. Sci.*, **36**, 1327–1335.

Maeda, N., Klyce, S. D., Smolek, M.K. and McDonald, M. B. (1997) Disparity of keratometry readings and corneal power within the pupil after refractive surgery for myopia. *Cornea*, **16**, 517–524.

Maguire, L. J., Singer, D. E. and Klyce, S. D. (1987) Graphic presentation of computer-analyzed keratoscope photographs. *Arch. Ophthalmol.*, **105**, 223–230.

Maguire, L. J., Zabel, R. W., Parker, P. *et al.* (1991) Topography and ray tracing analysis of patients with excellent visual acuity 3 months after excimer laser photorefractive keratectomy for myopia. *J. Refract. Corneal Surg.*, **7**, 122–128.

Maguire, L. J., Wilson, S. E., Camp, J. J. and Verity, S. (1993) Evaluating the reproducibility of topography systems on spherical surfaces. *Arch. Ophthalmol.*, **111**, 259–262

Maloney, R. K. (1999) Discussion: Posterior corneal surface topographic changes after laser in situ keratomileusis are related to residual corneal bed thickness. *Ophthalmology*, **106**, 409–410.

Maloney, R. K., Bogan, S. J. and Waring, G. O. (1993) Determination of corneal image-forming properties from corneal topography. *Am. J. Ophthalmol.*, **115**, 31–41.

Martinez, C. E., Applegate, R. A., Klyce, S. D. *et al.* (1998) Effect of pupil dilation on corneal optical aberrations after photorefractive keratectomy. *Arch. Ophthalmol.*, **116**, 1053–1062.

Naufal, S. C., Hess, J. S., Friedlander, M. H. and Granet, N. S. (1997) Rasterstereography-based classification of normal corneas. *J. Cataract Refract. Surg.*, **23**, 222–228.

Nichols, J. J., Marsich, M. M., Nguyen, M. *et al.* (2000) Overnight orthokeratology. *Optom. Vis. Sci.*, **77**, 252–259.

Olsen, T., Dam-Johansen, M., Bek, T. *et al.* (1996) Evaluating surgically induced astigmatism by Fourier analysis of corneal topography data. *J. Cataract Refract. Surg.*, **22**, 318–323.

Oshika, T., Klyce, S. D., Smolek, M. K. and McDonald, M. B. (1998a) Corneal hydration and central islands after excimer laser photorefractive keratectomy. *J. Cataract Refract. Surg.*, **24**, 1575–1580.

Oshika, T., Tomidokoro, A., Maruo, K. *et al.* (1998b) Quantitative evaluation of irregular astigmatism by fourier series harmonic analysis of videokeratography data. *Invest. Ophthalmol. Vis. Sci.*, **39**, 705–709.

Penney, C. M., Webb, R. H., Tiemann, J. J. and Thompson, K. P. (1993) Spatially resolved objective autorefractometer. United States Patent 5,258,791.

Rabinowitz, Y. S. and McDonnell, P. J. (1989) Computer-assisted corneal topography in keratoconus. *J. Refract. Corneal Surg.*, **5**, 400–408.

Riss, I., Hostyn, P., Kuhne, F. *et al.* (1991) Fiabilite et reproductibilite de photokeratoanalyseur de Nidek. *J. Fr. Ophthalmol.*, **14**, 451–454.

Roberts, C. (1994) Characterization of the inherent error in a spherically-biased corneal topography system in mapping a radially aspheric surface. *J. Refract. Corneal Surg.*, **10**, 103–111.

Rottenkolber, M. and Podbielska, H. (1996) High precision Twyman-Green interferometer for the measurement of ophthalmic surfaces. *Acta Ophthalmol. Scand.*, **74**, 348–353.

Rowsey, J. J., Reynolds, A. E. and Brown, R. (1981) Corneal topography. Corneascope. *Arch. Ophthalmol.*, **99**, 1093–1100.

Ruiz-Montenegro, J., Mafra, C. H. and Wilson, S. E. (1993) Corneal topographic alterations in normal contact lens wearers. *Ophthalmology*, **100**, 128–134

Seiler, T. and Quurke, A. W. (1998) Iatrogenic keratectasia after LASIK in a case of forme fruste keratoconus. *J. Cataract Refract. Surg.*, **24**, 1007–1009.

Seiler, T., Reckmann, W. and Maloney, R. K. (1993) Effective spherical aberration of the cornea as a quantitative descriptor in corneal topography. *J. Cataract Refract. Surg. (Suppl.)*, **19**, 155–165.

Shack, R., Baker, R., Buchroeder, R. *et al.* (1979) Ultrafast laser scanner microscope. *J. Histochem. Cytochem.*, **27**, 153–159.

Smolek, M. K. (1994) Holographic interferometry of intact and radially incised human eye-bank corneas. *J. Cataract Refract. Surg.*, **20**, 277–286.

Smolek, M. K. and Klyce, S. D. (1997) Current keratoconus detection methods compared with a neural network approach. *Invest Ophthalmol. Vis. Sci.*, **38**, 2290–2299.

Swinger, C. A. and Barker, B. A. (1984) Prospective evaluation of myopic keratomileusis, *Ophthalmology*, **91**, 785–792.

Warnicki, J. W., Rehkopf, P. G., Curtin, D. Y. *et al.* (1988) Corneal topography using computer analyzed rasterstereographic images. *Appl. Optics*, **27**, 1135–1139.

Wilson, S. E. and Klyce, S. D. (1991) Quantitative descriptors of corneal topography: A clinical study. *Arch. Ophthalmol.*, **109**, 349–353.

Wilson, S. E., Lin, D. T., Klyce, S. D. *et al.* (1990) Topographic changes in contact lens-induced corneal warpage. *Ophthalmology*, **97**, 734–744.

Wilson, S. E., Verity, S. M. and Conger, D. L. (1992) Accuracy and precision of the corneal analysis system and the topographic modeling system. *Cornea*, **11**, 28–35.

Wilson, S. E., Klyce, S. D. and Husseini, Z. M. (1993) Standardized color-coded maps for corneal topography. *Ophthalmology*, **100**, 1723–1727.

Yaylali, V., Kaufman, S. C. and Thompson, H. W. (1997) Corneal thickness measurements with the Orbscan Topography System and ultrasonic pachymetry. *J. Cataract Refract. Surg.*, **23**, 1345–1350.

Zadnik, K., Friedman, N. E. and Mutti, D. O. (1995) Repeatability of corneal topography: the corneal field. *J. Refract. Corneal Surg.*, **11**, 119–125.

Index

To promote excellence in contact lens research, manufacturing and clinical practice

Annual Clinical Conference
Annual Trade Exhibition
Continuing Education Courses
Contact Lens and Anterior Eye
(the Journal of the British Contact Lens Association)
Research Grants
Award Lectures

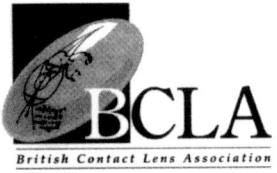

BCLA
British Contact Lens Association

Vivien Freeman, British Contact Lens Association, Walmar House,
288 - 292 Regent Street, London W1R 5HF, United Kingdom
Telephone number + 44 (0) 20 7580 6661
Fax number + 44 (0) 20 7580 6669
E-mail: vfreeman@bcla.org.uk • Website: www.bcla.org.uk

bringing the optical profession into focus

Butterworth-Heinemann and **Optician** have redesigned their international website

optometry online.net

- All the latest news updated as it happens
- Continuing Education and Training
- Fully searchable archive of Optician articles
- Columns from our international contributors
- The latest optometry jobs
- Letters and comment

- Butterworth-Heinemann's online bookshop
- A dictionary of optometric terms
- Improved directory of manufacturers, brands and professional associations
- General business news, weather and travel

PLUS more developments coming soon!

For a free optometryonline.net internet access CD-ROM call 0870 6012303*

- ☐ **FREE!** Internet access with free Internet Explorer 5™
- ☐ **FREE!** Fifteen email addresses @optometryonline.net
- ☐ **FREE!** 10 MB web space
- ☐ **FREE!** Online help
- ☐ **FREE!** Outlook Express software

*This offer is only available in the UK

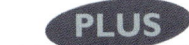 **BUTTERWORTH HEINEMANN** Optician

two leading names one leading site